Daisy Ch

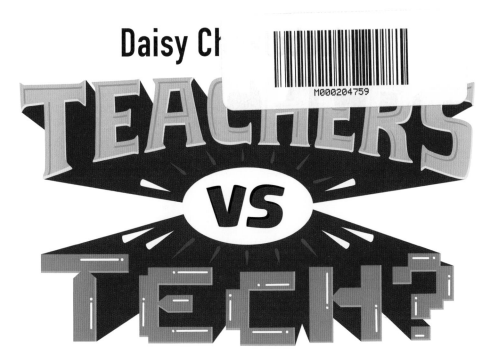

The case for an ed tech revolution

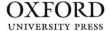

OXFORD

UNIVERSITY PRESS

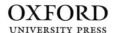

OXFORD

UNIVERSITY PRESS

Great Clarendon Street, Oxford, OX2 6DP, United Kingdom

Oxford University Press is a department of the University of Oxford. It furthers the University's objective of excellence in research, scholarship, and education by publishing worldwide. Oxford is a registered trade mark of Oxford University Press in the UK and in certain other countries.

British Library Cataloguing in Publication Data
Data available

ISBN 978-1-3820-0412-1

1 3 5 7 9 10 8 6 4 2

Typeset by Aptara

Paper used in the production of this book is a natural, recyclable product made from wood grown in sustainable forests.

The manufacturing process conforms to the environmental regulations of the country of origin.

Printed in Great Britain by Bell and Bain Ltd., Glasgow

Acknowledgements

The publisher and authors would like to thank the following for permission to use photographs and other copyright material:

All illustrations by Oliver Caviglioli (**p4, 5, 6, 13, 25, 32(t, b), 41, 43, 52, 65, 67, 95, 97, 107, 123, 125(t, b), 127, 129, 148, 149, 172, 173, 191, 193, 232**), except: **p15**: BECTA/OUP; **p7, p114(t, b), p182(t, m, b)**: OUP; **p90**: Oakley, B.A., Sejnowski, T.J. What we learned from creating one of the world's most popular MOOCs. npj Sci. Learn. 4, 7 (2019) doi:10.1038/s41539-019-0046-0/Creative Commons Attribution 4.0 International License.

Cover illustration by Risa Rodil.

Every effort has been made to contact copyright holders of material reproduced in this book. Any omissions will be rectified in subsequent printings if notice is given to the publisher.

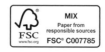

On two occasions I have been asked, — "Pray, Mr. Babbage, if you put into the machine wrong figures, will the right answers come out?" I am not able rightly to apprehend the kind of confusion of ideas that could provoke such a question.

Charles Babbage, *Passages from the Life of a Philosopher*

Contents

Foreword
by Paul Kirschner

They say that clothes make the person (*vestis virum facit*)[1]. In essence, this proverb means that people are judged according to the way they are dressed and not by who they are and what they do. But is this really true, especially when it comes to teaching?

Is it the teacher and what (s)he knows and can do that makes the difference? Or is it, as modern-day education often seems to imply, the technological window trappings that education has been bombarded with? In my humble opinion, and with respect to teachers, it's definitely the former.

I myself, a former cook and head of a restaurant, tend to use cooking as an analogy, so bear with me. Let's draw a comparison between teaching and cooking. Both are professions which, when carried out well, combine science with art and creativity. A top chef, and by this I mean a chef who is the creative director of a restaurant with a Michelin ranking, has a deep conceptual knowledge and has acquired very complex skills in relation to three things:

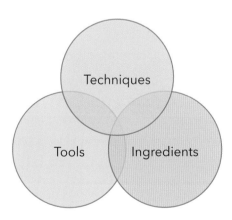

Top chefs have worked and learned for years and can perform magic in their restaurants. They plan, prepare and serve tasty, healthy and attractive dishes or meals to anyone, be they children, finicky eaters, diners with allergies or gourmands.

They can do this because they have deep conceptual knowledge and finely-honed skills with respect to the tools, techniques and ingredients (foodstuffs, plus herbs and spices) of their trade. A top chef knows when, how and why to use each tool, technique and ingredient, and also has the skills to use them to get the best results in any culinary situation. To do this they combine *science* (chemistry, physics, biology) with *art* to create meals that are healthy, good-looking and delicious.

In the same way, top teachers have worked and learned for years and can perform magic in their classrooms. They design, prepare and implement effective, efficient and enjoyable learning experiences for learners who are advantaged or disadvantaged, have special needs, who require additional or specific types of support, and so forth.

They can do this because they have deep conceptual knowledge and finely-honed skills with respect to:

- the tools of the teaching trade, from book and whiteboard through to advanced ICT

- pedagogy, in the sense of instructional techniques, from lecture through to project-based and collaborative learning

- ingredients, which include both domain-specific content as well as the different types of questions, prompts, tasks, examples, simulations, and so on.

A top teacher knows when, how and why to use each of their tools, techniques and ingredients, and also has the skills to properly implement them in different situations and with different students. To do this, they combine *science* (from educational, psychological and organizational sciences) with *art* and creativity to produce learning situations that are effective, efficient and enjoyable for their students and for themselves.

And just as top chefs don't begin with – nor base their cooking on – the newest kitchen tools or gadgets, top teachers don't decide what or how to teach based on the newest instructional hypes and technology trends.

To that end, what you will read in the rest of this book is an eloquent discussion of what top teachers need to know about technology and what it can and cannot do for teaching and learning. Daisy Christodoulou helps teachers – but hopefully also head teachers/principals, administrators, educational policy makers and even politicians – connect the dots between what good education is, the technology they have at their disposal and the research and evidence-base underpinning them both.

In other words, you will become empowered to make evidence-informed decisions around teaching and learning. As Daisy says herself, only then can we unlock the enormous promise for a genuine – and unexpected – revolution.

Until now we've had only two real revolutions with respect to teaching. The first was the printing press. As Daisy explains, before the invention of the printing press, books were extremely expensive and scarce. Only the rich were able to possess books and take heed of the information in them. With the advent of the printing press, and especially the printing press with moveable type, books became widely available, making a wealth of information (and also disinformation) available to many.

The second revolution was the blackboard (also called a chalkboard) at the beginning of the 19th Century. Before the blackboard, schools were primarily one-room buildings and 'following lessons' generally meant students worked on their own copying out texts. Schools were underfunded and one teacher might be responsible for hundreds of students. Steven Krause[2] writes that the blackboard was a revolution, in that it allowed teachers to work with large groups of students all at once. It also helped reduce the need to buy books, paper and ink. A blackboard, often made of slate (and hence the name) or a wooden board painted black, let students and teachers demonstrate writing or how to solve mathematics problems to a whole class. In other words, teachers were now able to convey information to large groups of students in an effective and efficient way.

In my working life as an educational psychologist and instructional designer (at the time of writing, over 40 years), I've had to suffer the prophesies and predictions of trend watchers, trend matchers, futurologists, corporations, educational gurus, and eduquacks telling me how information and communication technologies were the next revolution in education. Up until now, these technologies have been little more than expansions of the first two real revolutions.

Daisy ends her book as follows:

> … [I've] read many different explanations of why education technology has failed and what it would take to change that. If only there was more money, or better training, or more open-minded teachers, or schools that weren't designed to be like factories, then technology really could improve education.
>
> However, ultimately I have concluded that more important than any of these factors is the power of bad ideas. If we assume that learning styles exist, that cognitive overload doesn't exist, that students can pick up knowledge as they

go, and that attention is an infinite resource, we will never improve education, however much, or little, technology we use. If we persist with faulty ideas about how humans think and learn, we will just extend a century-long cycle of hype and disillusionment.

In other words, if clothes make the person, then with respect to the use of technology in education, the emperor very often has no clothes.

With the knowledge that you can and will gain from this book, you as a teacher, administrator, or policymaker will be able to help education evolve to a new and higher level and maybe even revolutionize, if not education as a whole, your own teaching.

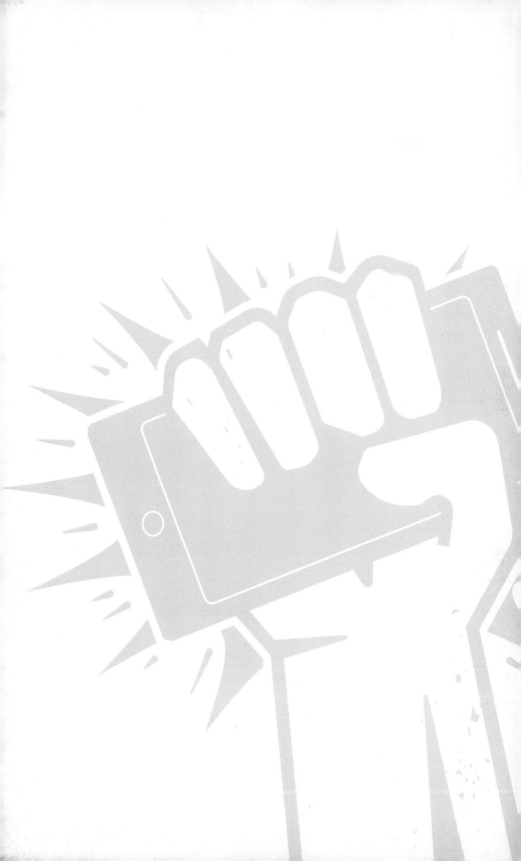

INTRODUCTION

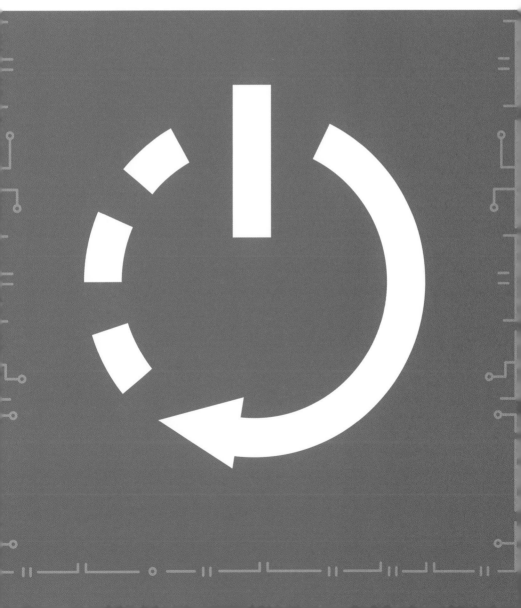

The history of the future

Books will soon be obsolete in the public schools. Scholars will be instructed through the eye. It is possible to teach every branch of human knowledge with the motion picture. Our school system will be completely changed inside of ten years.

Thomas Edison, quoted by Smith, F. J., 1913

People have been predicting that technology will transform education for over a century. And yet, with relatively few exceptions, education has remained untransformed. Books are not obsolete. The school system has not been radically changed in the way Thomas Edison predicted. Children still attend school buildings and sit at desks in ways that are similar to their counterparts in the 19th Century. Compared to the change and disruption that technology has brought to practically every other part of our society, education is an outlier.

This has not been for lack of effort – or money. Many developed countries have made big investments in education technology, but data from the Organisation for Economic Co-operation and Development (OECD) shows that these have led to 'no appreciable improvements' in educational achievement.[1] In developing countries, many big philanthropic technology projects have been similarly unsuccessful.[2–3]

Why is this?

I first got interested in this question when I began teaching in 2007. Although I had only left school myself four years earlier, those intervening years had seen huge investments in interactive whiteboards in English schools. I'd never seen an interactive whiteboard when I was a student, but by the time I started teaching they were in almost every state school in the country.[4]

England's investment in interactive whiteboards

England invested heavily in technology in schools from 1997 onwards. By 2002–3, the government was spending £510 million a year on its ICT in Schools initiative, and interactive whiteboards were an important part of this strategy.[5] In 2004, the then Education Secretary, Charles Clarke, announced a fund of £25 million for schools to purchase interactive whiteboards.[6]

It's estimated that in 2004, schools in England spent £50 million in total on interactive whiteboards.[7] The result was a dramatic increase in the number of whiteboards in classrooms, as can be seen from the graph below.[8]

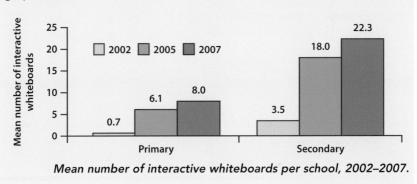

Mean number of interactive whiteboards per school, 2002–2007.

Viewed in isolation, these whiteboards seemed like magic. I remember the first time I saw one in action, I couldn't quite believe they were real. You could write on a whiteboard, have your words or diagram appear on the screen and on the linked computer, and then save all your jottings for a future lesson. Various different linked software packages and pre-planned lessons let you exploit the interactivity in different ways.

However, once I was in the classroom, despite my best intentions, I rarely used any of the most sophisticated features, instead using the whiteboard to display pre-prepared slides and presentations. I wasn't alone in this, one education academic lamented the way that teachers (like me) used interactive whiteboards as 'very expensive data projectors' and noted that:

> … in nine out of 10 schools I visit there is only one cable plugged into the teacher's laptop, and that is the projector. The whiteboard cable is out.
>
> Angela McFarlane, quoted by Lepkowska, D., 2007

However they were being used, they weren't having the hoped-for impact on attainment. One major review of their use concluded that:

> … although the [interactive whiteboard] may alter the way that learning takes place, and that the motivation of teachers and pupils may be increased, yet this may have no significant or measurable impact on achievement.
>
> Higgins, S., Beauchamp, et al., 2007

How could such a big investment in such cutting-edge technology end up producing such disappointing results? Speaking to colleagues and others in education, I would often hear variants of two arguments, neither of which I found satisfactory.

One was that teachers were conservative and change-averse and when they got new technology, they would default to using it in 'old' ways, like I had. This argument never felt very persuasive to me because I and my fellow trainees were new to the profession and not accustomed to any particular teaching approach. If we had ended up using whiteboards in traditional ways, it was not out of habit but because other methods had proved unworkable or unsatisfactory in some way. For example, a lot of the advice about how to use interactive whiteboards recommended giving individual students the chance to come to the front of the class and use the whiteboard themselves. But it often felt to me that doing this was not of as much value for the rest of the class, and indeed, a review of whiteboard use showed that these kinds of activities did lead to 'a loss of pace, and boredom of more able pupils.'[9]

The other argument I would hear is that education is immune to technology, that it's simply too 'human' or too 'personal' to allow for computers to have much of a role. This explanation never seemed that compelling either. Technology has a big role to play in other very human and personal areas like dating and healthcare. It felt unlikely to me that education was so unique that it could not be affected by technology. At least, if education really was the one area of human endeavour where technology could not have much of an impact, I would want more of an explanation than just 'it's too human'.

England's investment in interactive whiteboards has been described by a later government minister as an example of the government 'imposing unwanted technology on schools'.[10] Still, it was markedly more successful than some other high-profile and expensive projects, as we will see in the following case study.

Tablets in Los Angeles

In 2013, the Los Angeles Unified School District (LAUSD) announced a deal with Apple and Pearson (a leading educational publisher) to equip every student in the district with iPads that carried a Pearson curriculum.[11] The LAUSD is the second-largest school district in the US, educating over 700,000 students, and the contract would ultimately have cost $1.3 billion. Barely a year later, the deal collapsed. The iPads' security software was easy to delete, the pre-installed curriculum was unfinished and riddled with errors, and teachers had been given little training in how to use the tablets and curriculum.[12]

Perhaps the most chastening aspect of this failure was the stature of the organizations involved. As *Wired* magazine reported:

> If one of the country's largest school districts, one of the world's largest tech companies, and one of the most established brands in education can't make it work, can anyone?

Lapowsky, I., 2015

17

So why has education technology failed in the past, and is it destined to keep failing in the future?

This book will explore these questions and try to come up with some more nuanced answers than 'obstinate teachers' or 'education is special'. As we can see from Edison, making predictions is a dangerous game. It's easy to be overoptimistic and make predictions that don't come to pass. But it's also possible to be too pessimistic and dismiss good ideas.

A few years before Edison's prediction about books and film, many eminent scientists thought that human flight was impossible.[13] And indeed, in the 1890s, it probably would have seemed more likely that the new technology of radio waves could transform education than that passenger flight would transform travel. At around the same time, parapsychology and clairvoyance were burgeoning new fields of enquiry that seemed to have a promising future. Sometimes, popular, plausible and commonsensical ideas turn out not to have the impact we would hope for, whereas less plausible ones can be transformative.

It's easy to laugh cynically at new inventions, and it's equally easy to fall gullibly for them. As a result, deciding to be either 'pro-' or 'anti-' technology is not helpful. In this book, my aim is to move away from such dichotomies. Sometimes, I will be critical of popular and plausible arguments, but at other times, I will entertain ideas that seem more fanciful. I hope that by looking at the history of past education technology failures, at the nature of education, and at the way technology has succeeded in changing other fields, we can avoid some obvious errors and make success more likely.

This feels particularly urgent because over the past five years or so there has been a surge of interest in education technology, with a wealth of new approaches promising to make a difference. At the same time, the debate about the value of education technology has intensified, with almost as many viewpoints as education apps. Some teacher union leaders welcome investment in technology, while others fear it could reduce the need for teachers.[14–15] Some teachers feel it could reduce workload; others say it's increased it.[16–17] There are parents who worry about their children staring at screens all day, and those who worry that their children won't be able to get a job unless their schools embrace technology.[18–19]

Before we consider these competing arguments, let's take a step back and look more broadly at education in general. Regardless of technology, does education need to change? Is our current educational model fine, does it need tweaking, or is it in need of more radical upheaval?

Does education need to change?

The 20th Century saw a global expansion of primary and secondary education which brought with it many benefits. Children spend more of their time in school, and global rates of literacy have never been higher.[20–21] Still, in both developed and developing countries, challenges remain.

To get an insight into different countries' education systems, we can look at the data from Programme for International Student Assessment (PISA) tests. The PISA tests are run by the Organisation for Economic Co-operation and Development (OECD), and every three years they assess thousands of 15-year-olds in dozens of countries on their achievement in mathematics, science and reading. The results consistently show that even in developed countries, significant minorities have weak skills, which makes it hard for them to participate in modern society.[22–24]

In 2012, the OECD carried out a new assessment designed to measure adult skills, and also to compare different generations across time. In Korea, adults in the 55–65 age range performed poorly, but those aged 16–24 did much better.[25] But in England and the United States, 'improvements between younger and older generations are barely apparent'. This may partially be explained by historical reasons: many Korean adults in the 55–65 age range will not have had any formal education in the aftermath of the country's civil war. But that can't completely explain the lack of improvement in England and the US.

In developing countries, of course, lots of children do not even have access to education and those who do may not have access to quality education. The literature on global educational achievement often measures how many children are enrolled in school and for how long. Of course, it's important to know these statistics, but they can be misleading, because a year's worth of schooling in one country is not the same as a year in another. The education economist Eric Hanushek has shown that when you factor in educational quality, 'the education deficits in developing countries are larger than previously thought'.[26]

Other data shows some worrying patterns. Throughout the 20th Century, scores on IQ tests increased steadily, a phenomenon known as the 'Flynn effect' after the scientist who discovered it.[27] In recent years, there have been signs that the Flynn effect has stalled or even gone into reverse.[28] The reasons for the existence of the Flynn effect, and for its reversal, are not clear, and they may be the result of factors outside education.

However, this lack of understanding is part of the problem. We know relatively little about what makes good education and how we can reliably improve it. In other areas of life, such as economic growth or life expectancy, we are accustomed to seeing steady, if small, annual increases that add up to big differences over time. In education, that engine of improvement appears to be missing.

The OECD research cited at the beginning of this introduction showed that investments in technology don't lead to appreciable improvements in outcomes. Other research by the OECD shows that beyond a certain level, increasing general investment in education doesn't lead to improvements either: there is no clear correlation between spending per student and education outcomes.[29] And some of the most popular school-improvement tactics turn out not to have as much impact as you might think, either. Reducing class sizes, for instance, is beloved of politicians, but has limited impact on student attainment.[30] In Chapter 2, we will look more closely at why this is, and we will explore how different methods of more personalized instruction can support or impede student learning.

What will improve education?

Before we can think about using technology in education, or indeed making any expensive intervention, we need to step back and ask some broader questions. Much education research is focussed on describing the features of successful school systems. This can be interesting and useful in some ways, but it also has limitations. It is hard to know whether the prominent features of a particular system cause that system to be successful, or whether the causes of success are deeper and less visible. E. D. Hirsch, the educationalist, uses an analogy from medical science to make this point. Originally, medical researchers assumed that malaria was caused by damp, low-lying air, because many of the people who got the disease lived near swamps. Only later when the disease was put under a microscope did they discover it was transmitted through mosquito bites.[31] Similarly, with education, we need to think about cause and effect in a deeper way. Instead of just looking at the features of successful schools and school systems, we need to ask more fundamental questions: *how do humans learn*? and *what causes learning to happen?*

Once we have some answers to those questions, then we can start to think about *how* technology can help us achieve our educational goals. That's the aim of this book. In Chapter 1, we'll look at what the science says about how humans learn. Chapters 2–5 will each focus on a popular education technology strategy and see how it measures up against the science. Chapters 6 and 7 will then establish some principles for how technology can reliably help education.

Education technology is an enormous, global and fast-moving field, and this book is not an exhaustive survey of it or a catalogue of the best learning apps. Rather, when I discuss a particular programme, it's because it illustrates some general principles or illuminates a wider debate.

The focus of the book is on primary and secondary school education, with some diversion into tertiary education where there are signs an approach might transfer well to schools. I've looked at different approaches from across the world, but there is an inevitable bias towards the UK, the system I know best.

I have also deliberately focussed on the educational programmes of some of the major US technology companies and their charitable arms, simply because these organizations have enormous resources and global influence. Their general support for a particular approach is of significance, even when their specific interventions may be small and limited to the US.

One of the central themes in the book is the gap between what we know about human cognition, and what often gets recommended in education technology. In the last 70 years or so, scientists have discovered enormous amounts about how the human mind works. Much of this research has been inextricably intertwined with research into artificial intelligence and information technology, as researchers realized that to understand how to develop artificial intelligence, they had to understand how human intelligence worked.[32]

But while this research has led to the dramatic developments in technology which have transformed so much of our world, the same research is incredibly little-known in education. The greatest irony of all is that education technology has perhaps been the faddiest part of education. Far from establishing sound research-based principles, technology has been used to introduce yet more pseudoscience into the education profession. But therein also lies the greatest hope: if we can reconnect both education and technology with the research underpinning them both, there is enormous promise for a genuinely successful revolution.

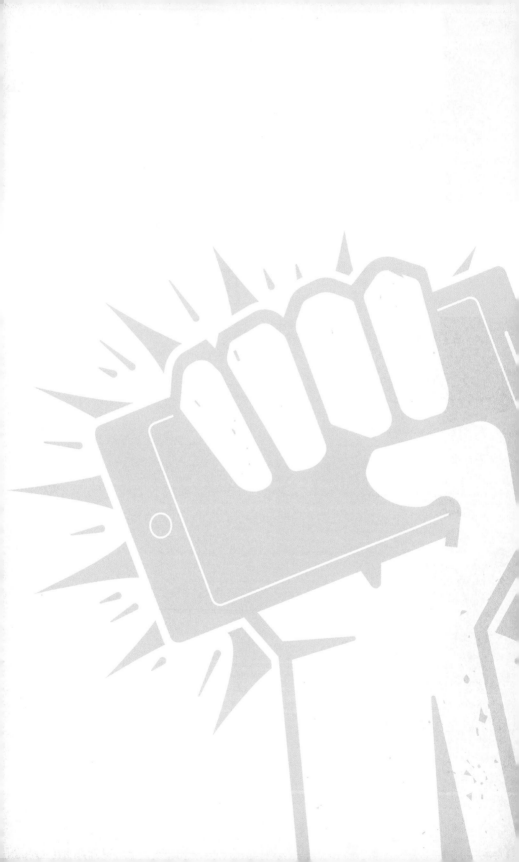

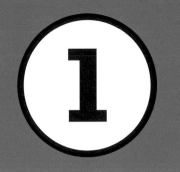

THE SCIENCE OF LEARNING

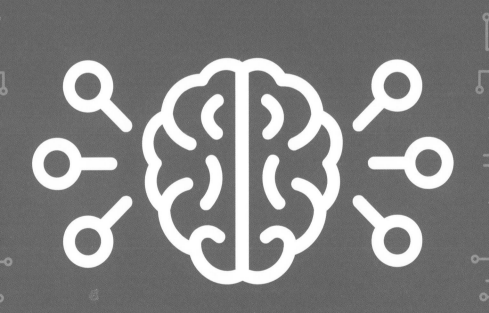

What causes learning?

What causes learning to happen? Many of us, whether teachers or otherwise, will have asked ourselves a version of this question. Why is it that we find some skills easy to pick up, and others resistant to lots of hard work? Why does some knowledge stick unwittingly in our memories, and some just drain away?

I had always been interested in these questions, but when I began teaching at an English secondary school in 2007, they assumed a new urgency. I came across constant examples of students' actions that were challenging to explain or rationalize. Once I asked a student to improve a piece of writing in which he'd used the word 'good' repetitively. He dutifully looked up 'good' in a thesaurus and returned with the sentence, 'I am a congenial footballer'.

With another class, I spent weeks preparing them for their GCSE English exam by practising how to 'read between the lines' and how to work out the meaning of words from context if they didn't know them. After a series of great practice lessons, they took a mock exam paper where they were all stumped by the presence of the word 'glacier', which none of them knew.

With other classes, I would mark sets of essays which would all routinely fail to use capital letters at the start of sentences. At the start of the next lesson, I'd ask the students what you should start a sentence with. Without fail, nearly all of them would chorus 'a capital letter!' 'Then why didn't you use one?', I'd say. At least they did remember the rule about a capital letter. With apostrophes, I could teach students an aspect of the how they are used one day and have them understand it by the end of the lesson. But then by the next lesson, some of them would have forgotten what an apostrophe even looked like.

Such experiences form the complaints of teachers worldwide, and they made up the substance of my complaints to my colleagues in the staff room. They are one of the reasons teaching is both fascinating and frustrating. I would teach students who were capable of razor-sharp insights when they spotted their teachers or parents behaving hypocritically, but who were unable to make the simplest inference about Pip's behaviour in the novel *Great Expectations*. They would remember off-the-cuff comments from me that I barely recalled saying, while forgetting the advice about exam structure that I nagged them about again and again.

What frustrated me the most was the inconsistency. Students would understand something one day, but not the next, and techniques that worked with one would fail with another. This inconsistency made it hard to tell if they were learning, and if my teaching was successful. Why did this happen? What could I do to help them apply their understanding consistently? Was it that they weren't trying hard enough, or that they lacked motivation or enough of a growth mindset? Or was it just that they were young, and that when they were a bit more mature, they could grasp such issues? These explanations offered some comfort, but they were never entirely satisfactory. Plenty of my students tried hard and were motivated. And lots of the older ones were still making the same mistakes, despite their more advanced years. There had to be a better explanation.

What I didn't realize then was that there was a great deal of interdisciplinary research which could explain these problems and which offered a way to solve them.

In the rest of this chapter we will look at this research. First, we'll look at some of the origins of this science of learning. Second, we'll look at one of its major insights, which is that all humans have a limited working memory and a vast long-term memory. Third, we'll look at more and less effective ways of getting information into long-term memory.

A science of learning

Perhaps the most fundamental and important principle is that there *is* a science of learning, and the existence of this science gives us some principles we can rely on regardless of who the student is. There *is* such a thing as a cognitive architecture which is common to humans. Of course, individuals will have particular differences, preferences and motivations, but those aren't the whole story. There are some universals which we can build on too, and they can be of enormous use to teachers, even if it doesn't mean that every student will respond in the same way to a particular teaching approach. Daniel Willingham, a cognitive scientist, explains it in this way:

> All students *do* have certain things in common. Indeed, it would be astonishing if they didn't. After all, we don't expect that individual human beings will differ radically in the way that the stomach participates in the digestion of food or the heart contributes to circulation. Why, then, shouldn't there be commonalities in the fundamental features of cognition, development, emotion, and motivation?
>
> Willingham, D. T. and Daniel, D., 2012

This might seem fairly obvious, but as we will see in the next chapter, there is much in education and education technology which is based on an entirely different reasoning: on the reasoning that students are very different, with different learning styles, and that we should attempt to group students into categories and teach to those learning styles instead. Unfortunately, despite the great popularity of the idea of learning styles, there is no evidence that they exist.[1] We'll look at this specific issue in more detail in Chapter 2.

Willingham's examples of digestion and circulation provide a useful analogy. Medicine is an applied science, and different humans react in different ways to the same treatment. Just because one person responds well to a drug doesn't mean that everyone will. However, the success and effectiveness of medicine have increased as we have learned more and more about biochemistry. We've established universal principles about the human body which inform medicine. Knowing the major human organ systems and how they work helps us to form hypotheses about which treatments might be more or less useful.

A science of how we think and learn could provide similar benefits for education. And establishing some universal principles can also help us think more clearly about the differences that do exist and that do matter. We will look at some of these differences in the next section of this chapter.

Where does this science come from?

Cognitive science is an interdisciplinary field which draws on research from different areas, including psychology, neuroscience, linguistics and computer science.[2] The history of these insights into human cognition are intertwined in fascinating ways with the history of modern information technology.

In order to create machines that can perform intelligent tasks, researchers tried to find out more about how the human mind works. And the invention of increasingly clever machines has, in turn, shed more light on how humans think.[3] A couple of examples will show this. One is a conference on artificial intelligence that was held in 1956 at Dartmouth University. The organizer, John McCarthy, coined the term 'artificial intelligence' (AI), and the conference is seen as the foundation of AI as a field of academic study.[4]

Attending the conference was Herbert Simon, who would win the Nobel Prize later in his career. Together with two colleagues, he presented the Logic Theorist, often called the first artificial intelligence program.[5] It was able to find proofs for many fundamental mathematical theorems and Simon saw the success of the project as 'launching the related disciplines of artificial intelligence and information-processing psychology.'[6]

Throughout the rest of his career, Simon remained interested in both human and machine intelligence, and, as we will see in Chapters 3–5, his research has huge implications for education. Also present at the conference was the psychologist, George A. Miller, who in that same year published a classic paper on the limitations of human working memory, which we'll discuss more in this chapter.

And that is not the whole story. The Logic Theorist has been superseded by approaches to artificial intelligence that are inspired by the neurons in human brains.[7] These neural networks have been at the forefront of some of the startling successes of AI over the last decade or so, such as facial recognition, self-driving cars and language translation. They work by recognizing patterns and learning from examples in the way that human brains do, and can provide some interesting insights into education too.

Working memory

The insight from the science of learning that perhaps has the most practical relevance for teachers is the distinction between working and long-term memory. Working memory 'is the small amount of information that can be held in mind and used in the execution of cognitive tasks'.[8]

You can test just how small an amount of information by giving yourself five seconds to look at the following 18 letters and memorize them all.

SBB CNH SGM TRA FIT VFA

Most people will find this task hard and will struggle to memorize more than about seven letters in total. This was the phenomenon George Miller identified in his 1956 paper, 'The Magical Number Seven, Plus or Minus Two'.[9] More recent research has expanded on Miller's findings, and suggested that working memory may be even more limited, to about four new items.[10] Working memory capacity does vary between individuals, and it also seems to be strongly connected with measures of general intelligence.[11] This is obviously one real difference between learners, one which most of us are familiar with.

However, this isn't the whole story. Working memory may vary, but it is still limited for everyone. If all we had to rely on when thinking was our working memories, then we wouldn't be able to do much thinking! As one group of researchers have said, given the intellectual feats that humans are capable of, it is likely that something other than working memory is being used.[12] In contrast to working memory, long-term memory is vast. Another quick test will reveal this. Give yourself five seconds to look at the following string of 18 letters and memorize them.

S BBC NHS GMT RAF ITV FA

Most British people will find this task much easier, even though the letters are exactly the same, and in exactly the same order, as the previous task. Why is it that people find the first task so hard and the second task so easy, when they are structurally so similar? The difference is that in the first task we are almost solely relying on working memory, which is easily overwhelmed. In the second, the letters have been organized so that they produce acronyms that will be familiar to most British people. With this task, we don't memorize the 18 letters as 18 individual items. Instead, we use the information we have in long-term memory to 'chunk' the 18 letters into more meaningful units. We're able to use the information we have in long-term memory to simplify the task.

Long-term memory, therefore, consists of elaborate and well-organized knowledge structures that provide us with a way of making sense of the everyday information we encounter.[13] Suppose we are reading a newspaper article and encounter the word 'money'. Most of us will have a well-developed knowledge structure that is automatically activated when we read the word 'money'. We might think of coins, credit cards, price tags and payslips. If we read the word 'bank' the sentence after reading the word 'money', then we are likely to think of financial institutions.

However, suppose we'd read the word 'bank' the sentence after reading the word 'river'. The knowledge structure we'd have called up from long-term memory would probably have been quite different.

One implication of this is that writers never set down exactly what they mean in complete detail. They are always leaving out more or less information for the reader to fill in from their long-term memory. To take a trivial example, imagine two different stories that begin with the following two sentences.

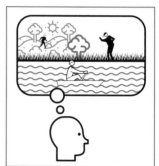

Bob stood in the lush meadows and listened to the sound of the boat's oars. John was standing by the bank.

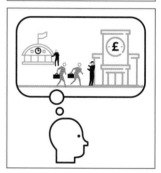

Bob stood outside the train station and watched the pinstriped financiers rushing by. John was standing by the bank.

The authors don't have to specify that in the first instance the bank refers to a river, and in the second to a financial institution. We can fill in that information ourselves – but only because we have knowledge about both riverbanks and financial banks.

We can also see from this that our minds work in an active way, seeking meaning and coherence, automatically supplying information that the writer has left out. When a typical reader reads those two sentences, they are adding all kinds of information from their long-term memory that help them to create meaning. We are not passive receivers of information: rather, we are active constructors of meaning.

We can perhaps appreciate this process more when it fails, as it will when we lack the relevant background knowledge. This is what happened, in the example I gave at the start of the chapter, to my students who were baffled by a short story about a glacier. They didn't know what a glacier was, and this prevented them from deriving meaning from the text. Compare that to a reader who *did* know what a glacier was: they could immediately access a rich mental structure of a threatening icy landscape which would have made sense of the short story.

This, in turn, shows us that another of the genuine differences between students which we should take account of in instruction is their prior knowledge, as that will determine their understanding of new knowledge. Differences in prior knowledge is one of the most significant differences between learners, and in many ways can be more significant than differences in general intelligence or working memory capacity.[14] We'll return to this theme again and again throughout this book in different contexts.

Prior knowledge also helps explain the differences between novices and experts. It's often easy to recognize expert performance when we see it. When someone reads a complex text and instantly makes an insightful inference, or looks at a chess board and selects a brilliant move, it's very impressive.

However, while it might be easy to recognize expertise, it's often harder to work out what causes it, and tempting to attribute it to superficial features. For example, we know that expert readers make fewer eye movements than beginner readers. So should we tell pupils who are learning to read to make fewer eye movements? No, because that might not be how expert readers learned to read.[15] Often, the way that you learn a skill is different from the way that you eventually use a skill. A great deal of research in a number of different areas suggests that the real causative and distinguishing feature between novices and experts is the extent and quality of the knowledge structures in long-term memory.[16] We'll look at this in more detail in Chapters 2–4.

The good news is that the differences between novices and experts, while real, are not immutable or fixed. A novice can become an expert by developing these knowledge structures. But how? What's the best method for doing so? Let's look at that next.

Building knowledge: minimal guidance vs direct instruction

Given what we have just seen about the importance of meaning-making, and the way our minds work in active ways, we might think that the best way to acquire these powerful structures of knowledge will involve some form of active enquiry and discovery, so that students can make the knowledge their own rather than have it passively drip-fed into their heads. And, given that we want our students to think like experts, we might want them to learn using the tasks experts use, and with less teacher guidance to stifle their thinking. A number of different approaches to teaching are based on these approaches.

Discovery learning and enquiry-based learning aim for students to discover insights for themselves. Project-based learning, hands-on activities and authentic tasks aim to present students with the types of unstructured activities they will encounter in the real world. We can sum up all of these approaches as being 'minimally guided', in that they all aim to reduce the guidance from teachers and give students the opportunity to construct their own meaning.

While minimally guided instruction might seem like a sensible way to help students construct meaning, in fact it has significant problems. Reducing guidance and structure makes tasks more complex, and complex tasks often overwhelm our limited working memories, making it hard for us to learn anything. A 2006 paper from the cognitive scientists Paul Kirschner, John Sweller and Richard Clark reviewed the evidence for minimally guided teaching and found that for novices, guided instruction is more effective because it reduces the load on working memory.[17]

The fundamental problem with minimally guided instruction is that it confuses the end goal of learning with the method of learning. It assumes that because we want students to be able to solve complex, real-world problems, the best way to achieve that aim is for them always to be solving complex, real-world problems. But to solve problems we have to acquire a lot of knowledge first. Acquiring these structures of knowledge is different from using them. Students do need to be mentally active in order to learn, but the mental activity must be directed in the right way.

What we need is a teaching method that requires high levels of mental activity, but where the mental activity is directed towards important features that are not too big to overwhelm working memory and that will help to develop long-term memory.

Direct instruction meets these requirements. It is interactive, but it still offers structure and guidance. In a direct instruction lesson:

> The teacher decides the learning intentions and success criteria, makes them transparent to the students, demonstrates them by modelling, evaluates if they understand what they have been told by checking for understanding, and re-telling them what they have told by tying it all together with closure.
>
> Hattie, J. 2009, p.206

Direct instruction involves lots of questions and answers, lots of review and repetition, and lots of opportunities for practice.[18] And the empirical evidence of its impact is strong. A 2004 meta-analysis of 12 direct instruction mathematics programmes showed positive results for 11 of them.[19] In John Hattie's 2008 educational meta-analysis, *Visible Learning*, direct instruction was one of the most effective approaches. A 2015 analysis of 13,883 first grade pupils in America showed that direct instruction helped them all to learn and was particularly valuable for those who had mathematical difficulties.[20]

One specific direct instruction programme is worth looking at more closely. DISTAR, the Direct Instruction System for Teaching Arithmetic and Reading, was the subject of one of the biggest and most famous education experiments in history, Project Follow-Through. The experiment studied over 200,000 children from kindergarten to grade 3 in America from 1968–77. The project compared the impact of different models of instruction and concluded that DISTAR produced the best outcomes for mathematics and reading, and that it had a positive impact on self-confidence too.[21] A 1996 follow-up study by Siegfried Engelmann and Gary Adams reviewed 37 more studies that showed a positive impact for similar programmes.[22]

One final piece of evidence is from the 2015 PISA study, which assessed the science achievement of 15-year-olds in 67 different education systems and compared the impact of teacher-directed instruction with enquiry-based instruction. The study found the following:

> In all but three education systems – Indonesia, Korea and Peru – using teacher-directed instruction more frequently is associated with higher science achievement.
>
> OECD, 2016, p.65

And:

> Greater exposure to enquiry-based instruction is negatively associated with science performance in 56 countries and economies. Perhaps surprisingly, in no education system do students who reported that they are frequently exposed to enquiry-based instruction score higher in science.
>
> Ibid., p.71

What about constructivism?

Another term that is frequently used in discussions of education is 'constructivism', which emphasizes the importance of students constructing meaning. While it's true that we do have to construct meaning for ourselves, that doesn't mean guidance is harmful. Structured approaches help us to construct meaning, whereas unstructured approaches can leave us confused. In a 2004 paper, educational psychologist Richard Mayer draws out the difference between these two senses of constructivism, calling them the constructivist view of learning and the constructivist teaching fallacy.[23]

Mayer accepts the constructivist view of learning: that 'learning is an active process in which learners are active sense makers who seek to build coherent and organized knowledge.'[24]

However, he does not agree that this means learners must discover everything for themselves. He calls this the 'constructivist teaching fallacy because it equates active learning with active teaching.'[25] He also notes that activities such as 'group discussions, hands-on activities, and interactive games' frequently get classified approvingly as 'constructivist', but they often promote not cognitive activity, but behavioural activity.[26]

The PISA 2015 study finds similar reasons to be concerned about 'hands-on activities':

> Activities related to experiments and laboratory work show the strongest negative relationship with science performance. While this correlational evidence should be interpreted with caution – for instance, teachers may be using hands-on activities to make science more attractive to disengaged students – it does suggest that some of the arguments against using hands-on activities in science class should not be completely disregarded.
>
> OECD, 2016, p.71

In Chapter 4 we will look in closer detail at different types of active learning, and how we can tell the difference between tasks that do and don't promote learning.

The cognitive science research also provides an explanation for the 'knowing-doing gap', the frustrating phenomenon where we know a rule, but fail to apply it reliably, like when students know that they should use a capital letter for proper nouns and at the start of sentence, but don't do so. Paradoxically, the knowing-doing gap is more likely if students are taught to write by 'doing writing'; that is, by practising writing stories, letters and lengthy articles with a 'real-world purpose'. These are exactly the types of task that can overwhelm working memory, because students have to think not just about all of the different technical aspects of writing, but also about the details of the topic they are writing about. By contrast, the specific practice that is a feature of direct instruction allows students to focus on a smaller skill, like starting a sentence with a capital, and practise it until it becomes a habit.

It is true that we can pick up some skills in an unstructured way. Children don't need explicit instruction to learn to speak and understand their mother tongue, for example. That's because learning to speak is a 'biologically primary' skill which we have evolved to develop quickly and easily.[27] But there are other 'biologically secondary' skills, like reading and writing, which we haven't evolved to develop in this way. Reading and writing are similar to speaking and listening, but they are not natural: they are inventions of late civilization.[28–29] Students do need to actively construct an understanding of good writing. But they're more likely to do this if the skill is broken down into manageable chunks and they are given guidance. We haven't evolved to decipher the mysteries of the apostrophe or sentence structure through unstructured exploration.

This also shows us why online search and digital reference sources are not the panacea they are often assumed to be. The knowledge we have stored in long-term memory is not a bolt-on part of cognition. It is integrated into all of our mental processes. When this knowledge is thoroughly integrated and fluent, it does not impose a burden on working memory at all. By contrast, looking something up on the Internet, or in any reference source, takes up valuable and precious space in working memory.

What's more, in order to look something up successfully, you need to have some idea both of what it is you are looking for, and what you expect to see. This may sound paradoxical, but consider the case of my student who used a thesaurus to change the sentence 'I am a good footballer' to 'I am a congenial footballer'. A research paper by George Miller, which explores exactly this phenomenon, concludes that while reference sources are great for people who already know a lot of words, they are not as effective as you might think as a means of learning new words.[30] We'll look at this in more detail in Chapter 3.

Education technology and cognitive science

Encountering this evidence from cognitive science was a bit like that moment in a detective novel when you finally realize 'whodunit' and why. These insights from research explained so much of the baffling behaviour of my students. As is often the case with a good detective novel, they also upended a lot of pre-existing stereotypes. Direct instruction had been one of those shifty characters lurking in the margins, exuding guilt. But the research suggested that it had been unfairly maligned, and those looking for a guilty party would do far better to look at enquiry learning, which had a spotless reputation during my training, but was suspiciously lacking in evidence.

The gap between research and education practice was the subject of my first book, *Seven Myths about Education*, where I showed the practical advice from education authorities in England was not supported by evidence. Since *Seven Myths* was published in 2013, English education has started to change for the better, partly because of shifts in policy, but also because many teachers are realizing the extraordinary explanatory power of cognitive science.[31]

However, I've also learned that a lot of the misleading approaches I encountered in my training in England are prevalent in many other parts of the world too. And education technology, despite its cutting-edge image, is often not much better.

In the next four chapters, we will explore the cognitive science research in more detail and look at how it applies to education technology.

- First, the personalization of learning: this is a popular idea right now, but given what the research on the science of learning shows, should we personalize instruction, and if so, how?

- Second, the fashionable slogan 'you can always look it up': surely the existence of powerful search engines and always-on smartphones means we don't have to worry as much about teaching facts?

- Third, active learning: we've already seen many different interpretations of active learning, so can technology help promote the more effective methods?

- Finally, what about those always-on devices: they clearly have the potential to be powerful aids to learning, but are they fulfilling it?

Summary

 There is a science of learning that can be applied to education.

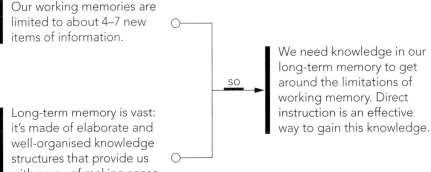

Our working memories are limited to about 4–7 new items of information.

Long-term memory is vast: it's made of elaborate and well-organised knowledge structures that provide us with a way of making sense of the everyday information we encounter.

SO

We need knowledge in our long-term memory to get around the limitations of working memory. Direct instruction is an effective way to gain this knowledge.

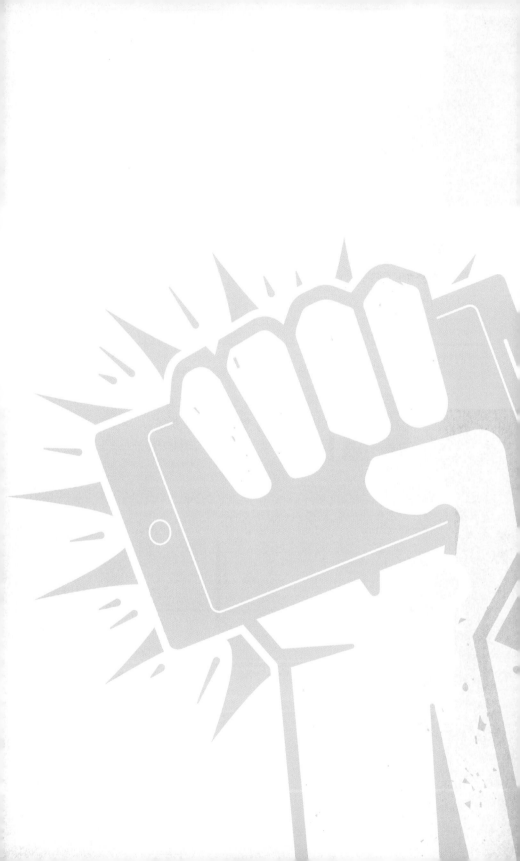

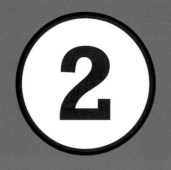

2

HOW CAN WE USE TECHNOLOGY TO PERSONALIZE LEARNING?

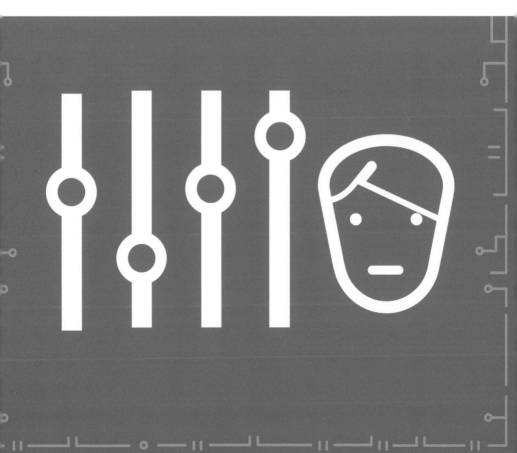

One teacher, many students

Most of us probably have memories of being in a class at school where we either struggled to keep up or were bored by how slowly the teacher was going. And most teachers will also have memories of teaching a class where it was difficult to meet the needs of every student. It's not hard to see why: traditional classrooms have one teacher and many children, so even if the teaching is excellent and the students are diligent, it is impossible for every student to receive instruction tailored precisely to their needs.

In Chapter 1, we saw that students do have a lot in common in the way they learn. However, one important and often overlooked difference is that each student brings different levels of background knowledge and vocabulary to the classroom. These can affect their understanding of quite straightforward concepts, and also mean that other differences can develop even over a short scheme of work on a new topic.

I can remember this exact problem when I taught the play *An Inspector Calls* to a group of 15-year-olds. At the beginning of the unit, they all knew very little about the play. But even with my best efforts, their understanding did not proceed in unison. After about ten lessons, I marked an assessment and realized that while a small handful of the students understood the play well, the majority of the class had confused two important characters. Meanwhile, one student had not taken the assessment as they had missed a series of lessons due to illness.

In an ideal world, I would have like to have cloned myself. I needed one version of myself to repeat the lessons for the absent student, another to explain the difference between Eric and Gerald, and another to teach the next lesson in the sequence. In the end I had to make some unsatisfactory trade-offs. Give the student who'd been ill a handout to read and work on; teach the rest of the class the difference between Eric and Gerald; and squeeze some of the next lesson's content into the remainder of the lesson.

Technology offers the promise of resolving these trade-offs, giving every student individualized instruction, assessment and feedback tailored to their precise needs. That's why personalization is one of the biggest buzzwords in modern education. Children have grown up choosing what they watch, what they hear, and what they see on their mobile phones. Perhaps the next step is to personalize their learning too, and perhaps the traditional 'one size fits all' classroom will soon look as outdated as TVs with one channel.

Can technology help give individualized instruction?

The technology entrepreneurs Mark Zuckerberg and Bill Gates have been enthusiastic about the potential of personalized learning: the Gates Foundation have invested $300 million into personalized learning approaches,[1] while Mark Zuckerberg has spoken in glowing terms of its potential on his blog, in an open letter to his newborn child.

> Our generation grew up in classrooms where we all learned the same things at the same pace regardless of our interests or needs.
>
> Your generation will set goals for what you want to become -- like an engineer, health worker, writer or community leader. You'll have technology that understands how you learn best and where you need to focus. You'll advance quickly in subjects that interest you most, and get as much help as you need in your most challenging areas. You'll explore topics that aren't even offered in schools today. Your teachers will also have better tools and data to help you achieve your goals.
>
> Even better, students around the world will be able to use personalized learning tools over the internet, even if they don't live near good schools. Of course it will take more than technology to give everyone a fair start in life, but personalized learning can be one scalable way to give all children a better education and more equal opportunity.

Zuckerberg M., 2015

Zuckerberg's charitable foundation, the Chan Zuckerberg Initiative (CZI), has backed this up with investments in various personalized learning projects too. In particular, they've funded the Summit Learning Program, an online personalized learning platform which is now being used in several hundred schools across America.[2]

Zuckerberg, along with many others, has cited a 1984 paper by Benjamin Bloom as proof of the value of personalized learning.[3] Bloom's paper showed that students who received one-to-one human tuition made gains of two standard deviations compared to those in traditional classrooms.[4] Two standard deviations is an extraordinary improvement. On a typical mathematics assessment, it's the equivalent of making eight additional years of progress in just one year.[5]

However, Bloom's paper does need some caveats. While other studies do show that one-to-one tuition can be effective, most do not tend to show such enormous gains.[6-7] This may be for a couple of reasons.

First, the students in Bloom's paper were being taught and assessed on completely new content on cartography and probability that none of them had ever studied before. Completely new content like this is very sensitive to instruction, meaning that students can make rapid gains over a short period of time. However, a lot of education research tends to focus on improvements on standardized tests in mathematics and reading. These types of tests are less sensitive to instruction, partly because the content isn't completely new, so prior attainment and knowledge will have a bigger impact.[8]

Second, Bloom's paper focussed on just a couple of hundred students in a few schools: large gains are more likely in small studies, and scaling up interventions generally tends to reduce their impact because it's difficult to maintain the fidelity of a programme across large numbers of teachers.[9]

For large-scale interventions measured with standardized mathematics and reading assessments, improvements of two standard deviations are unlikely, and an improvement of around 0.2 standard deviations is actually still impressive.[10]

Still, while two standard deviations may overstate the typical impact, one-to-one tuition is certainly effective. The challenge for personalized learning advocates is to find methods, often ones that use technology, that provide the benefits of one-to-one human tuition without the costs. However, this can then result in definitional problems, as many different approaches get bundled together under the heading of 'personalized learning' in the hope that something about them will reproduce the effect of one-to-one tuition.

For example, in 2017 RAND, the US research and development think tank, surveyed personalized learning and began by citing the Bloom paper. But it then acknowledged that 'there is not yet a widely shared definition of personalized learning' and went on to explore four very different strategies: learner profiles, personalized learning paths, competency-based progression and flexible learning environments.[11]

Similarly, a report by the UK Parliament in 2008 found it difficult just to define what personalization meant, let alone evaluate if it had been successful or not. The chair of the committee said that 'this is probably the most difficult inquiry that the Committee has undertaken since I have been the Chairman' and that 'a fog comes up' as soon as anyone mentions personalization.[12] Another member of the committee noted that a survey of 67 schools had identified more than 67 different interpretations of personalization.[13]

Given this, it would be extremely difficult to evaluate every possible interpretation of personalization. Instead, in this chapter I've picked out three distinct and relatively specific meanings of personalization, provided concrete technology-based examples for each, and considered how likely they are to improve learning given what we know about cognition.

These are:

1. Individual learning styles

2. Student choice

3. Adaptive learning

Individual learning styles

One popular interpretation of personalization is about tailoring instruction to the learning styles of individual students. A prominent advocate of this is Clayton Christensen, a business professor who is famous for developing the theory of disruptive innovation.

Disruptive innovation theory explains how technological innovations like the motorcar can disrupt and transform traditional industries. In his 2013 book, *Disrupting Class*, Christensen applies the same idea of disruptive innovation to education. For him, the great strength of technology is the way that it allows for personalization, and the best way to personalize instruction is with reference to the student's individual learning style. As he puts it:

> When an educational approach is well aligned with one's stronger intelligences or aptitudes, understanding can come more easily and with greater enthusiasm.
>
> Christensen, C.M., et al., 2010, loc. 616

Personalizing using learning styles

Christensen tells the story of a boy called Rob who struggles to understand how pressure operates on gases when it is taught using equations in the classroom, but who suddenly gets it when his father experiments with a balloon in the garage.

> Rob struggled to grasp the material when the teacher taught it in a logical-mathematical form. Almost surely this form of intelligence is not one of his strengths. His classmate, Maria, has a high logical-mathematical intelligence, so she grasped it immediately. But when his father demonstrated the same concept to Rob in a different, spatial way that aligned with how Rob learns, he not only understood, but found it interesting.
>
> Christensen, C.M., et al., 2010, loc. 616

Of course it would be difficult to provide this kind of personalized instruction in a typical school; the advantage of technology is that it could make video demonstrations like this available for all students who would find them helpful.

This interpretation of personalization is widespread, and similar to that given by the Summit Learning Program on their website:

> Think back to junior high — were you one of the kids who could read something once and retain it perfectly? Then lectures likely weren't as effective for you. Or maybe you excelled whenever you were able to do some project with your hands, which made every in-class video a snooze fest. No matter which student you were, finding out how to learn in the way that best fits *you* meant that you'd be able to really understand the lesson.
>
> Platt, K., 2019

The claim is clear. We all prefer to learn in a certain style, and when we are taught using that style, we will learn better. Maria needs to learn about pressure and gases with numbers and formulas, whereas Rob needs a visual demonstration. If you are teaching students a Shakespeare play, then perhaps some of them will learn best by reading it, some of them will learn best by watching a video of a performance, and others will learn best by acting it out.

This claim feels like it should be intuitively true, and many teachers think it is true.[14] However, it has been extensively researched, and consistently found lacking.[15–17] It is true that we have learning preferences.[18] That is, if asked, a student may well say that they would prefer to watch a video than to read a book. It is also true that we are better or worse at processing certain types of information.[19] That is, some students are better readers than others, and others are better at spatial reasoning.

However, the learning styles theory claims more than this. The learning styles theory doesn't just claim that we have a preferred style, or a best style. It claims that if we are taught in our preferred style, we will learn better. And that is not the case. **When we are learning, what matters most is not our preferred or best learning style, but the best learning style for the *content*.**[20]

Some content lends itself to particular modalities. If you want students to learn the locations of countries on a map of Africa, then a visual presentation of the material will be best. But the visual presentation of the material will be best for all students, *regardless* of their preferences or aptitudes. It would be unhelpful if you gave a map to the 'visual learners' and then read out loud a description of the map to the 'auditory learners'.

Similarly, while some material lends itself to being presented visually, other material does not, as Willingham explains.

Different representations are more or less effective for storing different types of information. Visual representations, for example, are poor for storing meaning because they are often consistent with more than one interpretation: A static image of a car driving on a snowy hill could just as well depict a car struggling up the hill or slipping backwards down the hill. And some concepts do not lend themselves well to pictures: How would one depict "genius" or "democracy" in a picture? On the other hand, the particular shade of green of a frozen pea would be stored visually because the information is inherently visual.

Willingham, D. T., 2005

Some material may benefit from being presented in more than one way. If we think back to Rob and Maria learning about gases, it may well be that both the presentation of the formula and the demonstration with the balloon were useful: but if they were useful, they would have been useful for both students.

Similarly, if a student is learning about Shakespeare, it would be useful for them to read the play, watch a performance of it, and act it out. It would be unfair if the only students who got to see plays were those who had been identified as 'visual learners'!

Plenty of research shows the value of combining words and images together.[21] For example, read the following text and try to answer the questions about it.[22]

Jenny is head of the Humanities faculty. Fatima is head of the History department. Tom, Joe and Sue work for Fatima. Harry is the head of the Geography department. Jo, Chaz and Tania report to Harry. Sue, Jo, Chaz and Harry are working together on the joint Modern Europe project.

1. Who is the highest-ranking person on the Modern Europe project?

2. Which department has the most people on the Modern Europe project?

3. Which people are not involved with the Modern Europe project?

Now look at the following combination of words and images, and try and answer the same questions.

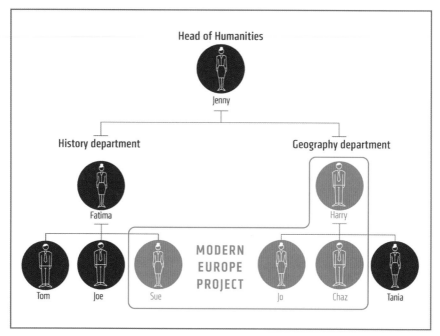

Organization chart revealing the value of combining words and images.[23]

The combination of words and images is easier to understand. But it's easier to understand for everyone, not just for learners with one particular learning style. And it consists of a combination of words and images, not words or images in isolation.

From this, we can see two ways in which the learning styles theory is not just false but actively unhelpful. First, it stops some students from receiving useful instruction, like a well-organized diagram of a mathematics problem or a combination of words and images. We shouldn't deny such resources to some students because 'it's not their style'.

Second, learning styles theories can create unhelpful stereotypes. As one literature review says:

> Many practitioners who use [learning styles] instruments think in stereotypes and treat, for instance, vocational students as if they were all non-reflective activists... Similarly, students begin to label themselves; for example, at a conference attended by one of the reviewers, an able student reflected – perhaps somewhat ironically – on using the Dunn and Dunn Productivity Environmental Preference Survey (PEPS): 'I learned that I was a low auditory, kinaesthetic learner. So there's no point in me reading a book or listening to anyone for more than a few minutes'.
>
> Coffield, F., et al., 2004, p.137

By encouraging students to focus on an initially mild preference or aptitude, we may end up limiting the types of concept they learn. That's the problem with the following advice from Summit Education:

> Once a student has found the best way to learn, the flexibility of every personalized learning classroom allows students to put that idea into action. This means, after a lecture or classroom discussion, different students within a single class could be completing different projects about the topic, each tailored to their learning style.
>
> Platt, K., 2019

The risk is that students who struggle with reading, but like watching films, will be actively encouraged to avoid reading and to focus on watching films instead. Students who enjoy reading will be encouraged to focus on written explanations solely, even though plenty of mathematics and geography problems are clearer when represented as an image or a diagram. Important skills and content that are particularly suited to one modality will become harder to learn for students who don't prefer that modality.

We think that translating material from one learning style to another will help a struggling student, but it can make it harder for them to learn.

Suppose a student does have a weaker aptitude for learning from images than other students. Suppose that weaker aptitude is interpreted to mean that they are 'not a visual learner' and so need to have maps described in words to them rather than seeing the image. Ultimately, this will just give them less practice with maps, making it harder for them to improve at reading maps.

Another example from Clayton Christensen's book demonstrates this problem. He retells an anecdote about a student who struggled to learn to read:

> When she entered the sixth grade, she had a teacher who observed how gracefully she moved, which prompted the teacher to wonder if she might learn through movement. Without being an expert in intelligence typologies, that teacher could see that this student had the gift of great bodily-kinaesthetic intelligence. The student generally refused to read, write, or practice spelling. But following her hunch, the teacher suggested to the girl that she "create a movement alphabet using her body to form each of the twenty-six letters." The next day, the girl ran into the classroom before school started with something to show her teacher. She danced each letter of the alphabet and then sequenced all twenty-six into a unified performance. She then spelled her first name and last name through dancing. That night she practiced all her spelling words through dancing—and performed the dance for her classmates the next day. Soon she began writing more and more words. First she would dance them; then she wrote them down. Her writing scores increased, as did her self-confidence. A few months later she no longer needed to dance out words to spell them; learning through her strength in bodily-kinaesthetic intelligence had opened a world of reading and writing to her forever.
>
> Christensen, C. M., et al., 2010, loc. 629

Is it really possible to use the strength of dancing to substitute for the weakness of reading in this way? The evidence suggests it cannot: 'Different memory representations store different types of information, [so] you usually cannot use one representation to substitute for another.'[24] Learning to read and write involves many different aspects, not all of which lend themselves well to kinaesthetic representation. Among other things, students have to learn the letters of the alphabet, the correspondences between groups of letters and sounds, how those different groups of letters can be combined to make words, and what those words mean. Expecting a struggling reader to solve their difficulties through dance risks leaving other serious issues undiagnosed and untreated.

Rather than providing students with instruction exclusively in the style that is supposed to appeal to them, we should instead be looking at the specifics of the content they are studying, as well as at more universal research-backed principles about how we manage information. In the next chapter, we will look more closely at the multimedia principle, which recommends that text, images and spoken words should be combined in particular ways for the best effect, and that doing so will have benefits for all learners.

Clearly, individual learning styles are just one interpretation of personalization. Let's explore some of the other ways that learning can be personalized.

Student choice

Another interpretation of personalized learning gives students more choice over the content they study and how long they study it for. The RAND survey of personalization in US schools that we looked at earlier discusses the advantages and disadvantages of students working in a 'self-paced environment' and finds that over half of the students in its sample get to choose the topics they study and the materials they use at least some of the time.

This type of personalization is also a part of the Summit Learning Program. What Summit call 'self-direction' is one of the three essential pillars of the programme.[25] In practice, this means students 'work at their own pace'[26], and 'take assessments when they feel ready, not at the same time as the rest of the class.'[27] In case studies on the Summit website, one student says that:

> As a Summit Learning student, the speed I learn depends on how I think and how quickly I understand the content.

Hill, I., 2018

A teacher reflecting on the programme says:

> Now when they go into the Platform, they choose how they want to best learn it, so one student might be watching a video, and somebody else could be taking PowerPoint notes. I think that choice and the personalized portion of the Platform really helps with engagement overall.

McNeil, K., 2018

We can see why this is an attractive proposition: in a traditional classroom, students can get bored or lost by the pace. Teachers can only devote a fraction of their time to each individual student. They can never know, minute-by-minute, how each student is doing, and even when they are aware a student is struggling or bored; they often cannot do much about it without disrupting the learning of lots of other students. By contrast, the student knows better than anyone how they are feeling about the material they are studying, and so will be better placed to make decisions about how to learn.

However, when we look at the research literature, it shows that often learners are not well-equipped to make good decisions about their learning, precisely because they are still learning. This is a specific example of the differences between experts and novices which we looked at in the previous chapter. One seminal paper in this field is by two researchers, David Dunning and Justin Kruger, whose findings have become known as the Dunning-Kruger effect.[28]

Student self-assessment – the Dunning-Kruger effect

The paper's central finding is that to make good decisions about our own competence in a particular area, we need to already possess a degree of competence in that area. If we don't have this baseline of competence, we often don't realize our weaknesses.

> The skills that enable one to construct a grammatical sentence are the same skills necessary to recognize a grammatical sentence, and thus are the same skills necessary to determine if a grammatical mistake has been made.
> In short, the same knowledge that underlies the ability to produce correct judgment is also the knowledge that underlies the ability to recognize correct judgment. To lack the former is to be deficient in the latter.
>
> Kruger, J. and Dunning, D., 1999

Dunning and Kruger carried out a series of experiments which demonstrate this. In one of them, they asked a group of undergraduates to take a grammar test and then, after they had completed the test, to estimate both how many questions they had got right and how well they had done compared to their peers who also took the test.

Lower-performing students significantly overestimated how well they had done on the test. They thought they had got 13 questions out of 20 right, when they had only got 9 right. They also thought that they had scored in the top third of all the students taking the test. But actually, they were in the bottom quarter. Dunning and Kruger repeated the study with tests of logical reasoning and humour, and found similar results.

In practice, teachers see this effect all the time, and it is one of the main reasons we need teachers. Take the story that I opened this chapter with, about my students confusing two characters in the play, *An Inspector Calls*. They hadn't made that mistake just to spite me: they really were genuinely confused about the two characters! If I had asked them to judge their performance on their essays, they would probably have thought they had done quite well. If they had been given the control over their own learning, they may well have chosen to move on to the next lesson in the unit, unaware of the significant error that was going to continue to impede their studies.

Other research backs this up and demonstrates more generally that our emotions and opinions are often not a reliable guide to learning. We may feel that repeating an easy task over and over again is boring, and not helping us to learn. Sometimes that is true, but sometimes, 'overlearning' in this way can be valuable, as it builds fluency and automaticity.[29] We can struggle when learning something for the first time, and think that is a sign we should stop or slow down. Again, that may or may not be right: 'desirable difficulties' are a part of learning, and judging just what makes a difficulty desirable or undesirable is often not easy.[30] In Chapter 4, we will look more closely at the types of activities which promote such desirable difficulties.

When it comes to revision, students' most popular strategy is to reread their notes. But this is one of the most ineffective strategies: self-quizzing is far more effective.[31] We can feel totally confident in our understanding of a topic and feel ready to move on. But we could just be deceived by familiarity, and we might need a lot more practice before we have understood it securely enough to tackle the next topic.[32]

Other research focusses even more specifically on the effects of giving students control over their own learning in hypermedia environments.

In this context, hypermedia refers to a mixture of images, text and hyperlinks where the student gets to choose what to read or click on next. One review of the available evidence by Katharina Scheiter concludes with the following: 'these reviews and meta-analyses provided highly consistent conclusions in that none of them found convincing evidence in favor of giving learners control over their instruction.'[33] One of the major reasons for this is that taking control of your learning is hard. It imposes a cognitive load that can distract from what you are trying to learn.[34]

The RAND paper on personalization shows some of the negative effects that can occur when students are given too much control over their learning:

> According to teachers, many students did not know how to organize their time so they would complete their work at a sufficient pace. For example, at the end of the second semester some students still had not completed work they were expected to do during the first semester.
>
> Pane, J. F., et al., 2017, p.18

It's easy to conclude that these students were being lazy or were simply not motivated, but they may just have lacked background knowledge on the topics they were studying, which in turn would have made it hard for them to plan how much time they would need to complete a topic. In the words of Scheiter's meta-review, 'learners with less prior knowledge have more difficulty navigating hypermedia systems, process information more superficially, and require more instructional support than their more knowledgeable counterparts.'[35]

Overall, the research on the importance of background knowledge for successful learning in a hypermedia environment makes an allied point to that of Dunning and Kruger. Dunning and Kruger show that lack of understanding makes it harder for a student to recognize their lack of understanding. The hypermedia research shows that the lack of understanding leads to people being overwhelmed when presented with choices.

One obvious and effective way of solving this problem is to increase a student's knowledge: that is, to teach them something. In the final study reported in their paper, Dunning and Kruger try exactly this. They gave the bottom-quartile students a set of tasks designed to teach them about the logical reasoning test they had performed poorly on. When the students completed these activities, their self-judgement improved dramatically.

Thus, Dunning and Kruger conclude that the way to improve judgement of your competence in an area is to improve your competence. Scheiter also finds that giving more knowledgeable students control over learning is useful and does lead to good choices being made.[36] Rather than expecting students to make good learning choices when they are novices, we should look at ways we can provide them with the guidance, structure and knowledge that will eventually allow them to make good learning choices.

Adaptive learning

So, the research shows that the most crucial differences between students may be to do with prior knowledge, not learning styles. And it suggests that the student's subjective opinion may not be a reliable guide to identifying such differences. The need for personalization remains, it's just that we should base it on accurate assessment of genuine differences. This is similar to how it works in other fields. Personalized medicine does not mean patients have to make their own diagnosis; rather, it is when clinicians make a diagnosis by using richer and more sophisticated data about the patient.[37] Similarly, personalized data can help teachers and students make better decisions about what each student needs.

This kind of personalization has a fairly long history, and it goes under some different names. In the late 1960s and 1970s, the first Intelligent Tutoring Systems were developed, which were designed to provide different questions and feedback to students based on their responses.[38] Over the last decade or so, the term 'adaptive learning' has more commonly been used to describe similar approaches. Here's a definition from Pearson, a leading educational publisher:

> Adaptive learning tools collect specific information about individual students' behaviors by tracking how they answer questions. The tool then responds to each student by changing the learning experience to better suit that person's needs, based on their unique and specific behaviors and answers.
>
> Edsurge, 2016, p.16

Rather than handing over control of learning to the student, these systems try to mimic what teachers would like to do if they had unlimited time and attention. Take my example of teaching *An Inspector Calls:* an adaptive system might ask all students a question like: Which character is the father of Eva Smith's baby? If one student incorrectly answers 'Gerald', then the programme could assign a video replaying a scene from the play, a short activity requiring them to explain the meaning of some key quotations in their own words, and then a further set of questions to test whether they had corrected their misconception. If another student gets the question right, that student would move on to a different sequence of activities.

Adaptive systems can also provide students with hints and tips in the way a teacher might, as the following example from a paper by Kurt VanLehn will demonstrate.[39]

Example of an adaptive digital teaching system

Suppose a student is given the question 2 + 3*x = 20, and asked to write the first step of the answer. Suppose they put: 5*x = 20. The system can then provide them with a series of hints, starting quite generally.

You seem to have added 2 + 3. Is that really appropriate?

If that doesn't work, the system can provide further information, and even give the student a simple, more constrained choice of whether to review a previous lesson or not.

Because multiplication has a higher precedence than addition, you should group 2 + 3*x as 2 + (3*x). If you want to review precedence, click here.

And if that still doesn't work, the system can provide the correct next step.

You should enter 3*x = 20 − 2.

The most complex and powerful adaptive systems build a model of both the subject being taught, and each individual student's understanding of it.[40] They will adapt what a student sees based not just on their response to the most recent question, but on their responses to past questions too. ALEKS is an adaptive system that models all the possible knowledge states within a topic like algebra, uses diagnostic questions to work out where a student's 'knowledge state' is, and then provides the right topic and questions to be studied based on this information.[41] Cognitive Tutor, one of the earliest and most popular Intelligent Tutoring Systems, was developed by the cognitive psychologist John Anderson and based on a broader theory of cognition.[42]

These systems are capable of providing different pathways through content for every student, with billions of possible knowledge states, and banks of hundreds of thousands of questions that can be accessed in a different order. Another example from an Indian programme, Mindspark, shows how adaptive systems can probe for misconceptions and offer follow-up activities to address this misconception:

> Mindspark examines patterns of error to target "differentiated remedial instruction." So if a student makes a mistake on which decimal is bigger (3.27 or 3.3), it may be due to "whole number thinking" (27 is bigger than 3) whereas if they make the same mistake with 3.27 or 3.18, it's probably "reverse order thinking" (comparing 81 to 72 because the "hundredth place" should be bigger than the "tenth place"). Mindspark then targets activities based on the likely reason for the mistake. A good teacher may catch this if most of the class is making the mistake, but it's much less likely if only a few students are making it. Those students get left behind.
>
> Muralidharan, K., et al., 2019

The evidence in favour of such programmes is fairly positive, although not completely consistent. A 2017 survey analysed 29 different programmes and concluded that 20 of them had a positive impact.[43] A 2014 meta-analysis looked at the impact of Intelligent Tutoring Systems in different subjects, different age ranges, and different countries. It found that in primary and secondary schools, they outperformed classroom instruction, and were about as effective as one-to-one tuition.[44] By contrast, a 2013 meta-analysis of primary and secondary mathematics Intelligent Tutoring Systems found that they had at best a small positive impact compared to normal classroom instruction.[45] A 2011 survey showed big improvements equivalent to those of one-to-one human tuition, but this combined school and university studies, and also featured some small-scale studies of new content which, as we've seen, are more likely to lead to big improvements.[46] Two major reviews of primary and secondary mathematics and reading programmes by Johns Hopkins University both showed a small positive impact.[47–48]

One challenge identified in the literature is how such systems should be used: whether they should replace classroom instruction completely, be integrated with classroom instruction, or only used as a separate homework programme. VanLehn outlines some of the challenges with each model: he notes that the process of building an adaptive system often leads to changes in the traditional way of teaching content. As a result, convincing teachers to adopt it can be difficult. He describes the approach of one Intelligent Tutoring System which aims to be part of a broader reform of the way instructors teach:

> They sell a whole curriculum that is consistent with recommendations from national panels and incorporates instruction developed by award-winning teachers... However, getting instructors and institutions to adopt curricular reforms is notoriously difficult, with or without an accompanying tutoring system. Scientific evidence of greater learning gains is only part of what it takes to convince stakeholders to change.
>
> VanLehn, K. et al., 2005

VanLehn's solution to this problem was to design a university physics course, Andes, that could be used for homework practice regardless of the precise way the actual course is being taught. Some school-level systems take a similar approach and are designed for school-age students to use at home, regardless of how mathematics is being taught in their school.[49] We'll explore the challenges of exactly how such systems should be used further in Chapter 6.

Adaptive systems are not perfect. They can be expensive and time-consuming to develop, and it's not clear they can capture everything that's involved in learning.[50] Currently, most adaptive systems designed for use in school are for mathematics and reading, not other curriculum subjects.[51] Still, they definitely have potential and the research clearly indicates that they are a far more effective way of personalizing education than learning styles or student choice.

Perhaps the biggest strength of adaptive personalized instruction is its focus on the details of instruction, the tricky bits of content that students often struggle with. Misconceptions like these can sometimes seem fairly trivial, but they compound and, if left uncorrected, can leave a student struggling with many other concepts. This attention to the detail of curriculum content is one of the major strengths of adaptive programmes. We'll explore this further in the next chapter, where we will look at different ways of providing curriculum content.

Summary

We can use technology to personalize instruction. But what's the best way?

We can personalize based on a student's preferred learning style.

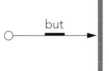
but

When we are learning, what matters most is not our preferred or best learning style, but the best learning style for the content.

We can personalize based on a student's choices and self-assessments.

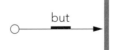
but

Novice learners struggle to identify their own strengths and weaknesses.

We can personalize based on insights from adaptive learning platforms.

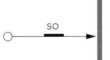
so

This allows us to focus on the details of curriculum content and instruction, making it possible to spot misconceptions.

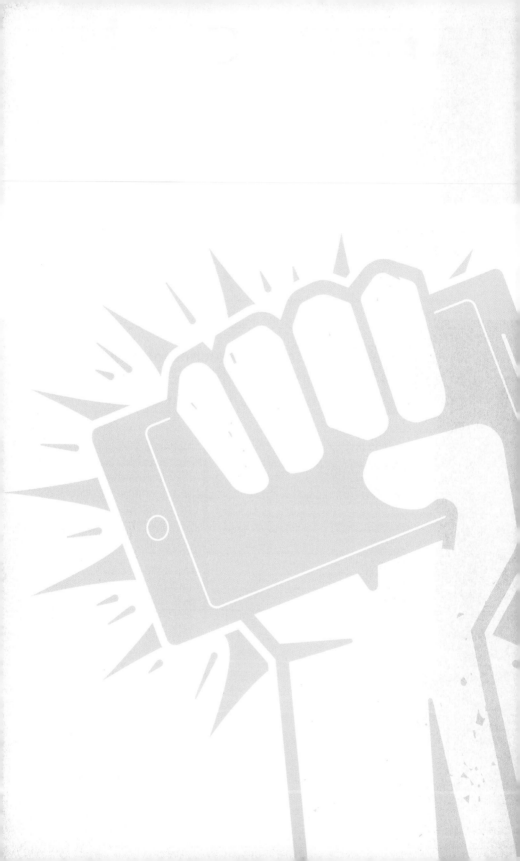

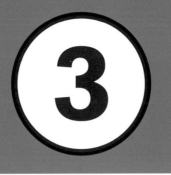

3

WHY CAN'T WE JUST LOOK IT UP?

Looking it up

One summer in the early 1990s, I can remember having a lengthy argument with my father about whether the children's author Richmal Crompton was a man or a woman. My father, a fellow fan of her writing, told me that when he was a little boy, he had thought 'Richmal' was a man's name. But when he was older he had read an article about her and discovered she was a woman. I was not convinced. Richmal sounded like a man's name, and in any case the books were about a boy, so they must have been written by a man. My father pointed out that plenty of women wrote books about boys and men. I pointed out that plenty of men wrote books about boys and men.

On and on it went. I was so persistent that my father started to waver. Perhaps he had misremembered? Maybe he had grown up assuming Richmal was a woman, and then read an article discovering he was a man? The reference sources we had at home were not that helpful. The local library had plenty of books by Richmal Crompton, but not much about her. We continued in this state of uncertainty for what felt like years. Eventually, my father stumbled across a short article about her in a Sunday newspaper – and yes, it turned out she was a woman. I remember poring over the piece of newsprint wondering if it could have been faked in any way.

We are probably the last generation who will ever have arguments like this. Today, a similar debate would be settled in seconds by using an Internet search engine. The Internet has transformed our access to all kinds of information: we can look up facts in a second, download entire books to our phones and ask questions of people on the other side of the world. These innovations have already changed the world of work, and so it seems only natural that they should change the world of education too.

One plausible suggestion is that, as information technologies make accessing knowledge cheaper and easier, schools should place less emphasis on knowledge and memorization. This is recommended by many major Silicon Valley leaders and thought influencers. Here is Marissa Mayer, CEO of the Internet company Yahoo:

> The Internet has relegated memorization of rote facts to mental exercise or enjoyment.
>
> Mayer, M., 2010

Here is Don Tapscott, technology author and a leading authority on the impact of technology on business and society:

> Teachers are no longer the fountain of knowledge; the internet is. Kids should learn about history to understand the world and why things are the way they are. But they don't need to know all the dates. It is enough that they know about the Battle of Hastings, without having to memorise that it was in 1066. They can look that up and position it in history with a click on Google.
>
> Don Tapscott, quoted by Wardrop, M., 2008

And here is Jonathan Rochelle, head of education apps at Google, discussing why children don't need to learn the quadratic equation anymore:

> I don't know why they can't ask Google for the right answer if the answer is right there.
>
> Jonathan Rochelle, quoted by Singer, N., 2017

Google

Google are perhaps a good place to start in this chapter, because the idea of 'Just Googling it' has become shorthand for the idea that we no longer need to know anything. Not only that, but out of all of the big technology firms, Google have arguably had the biggest impact on the classroom. According to Google's own 2019 figures, 30 million students and teachers worldwide use Chromebooks, and 40 million use Google Classroom, a classroom management tool that lets teachers and students share work and comments.[1]

Google also provide free resources, lesson plans and a teacher certification programme that's been completed by educators in 50 different countries.[2–3] A *New York Times* article in 2017 noted that in the United States:

> Google is helping to drive a philosophical change in public education — prioritizing training children in skills like teamwork and problem-solving while de-emphasizing the teaching of traditional academic knowledge, like math formulas.
>
> Singer, N., 2017

A major focus of Google's lesson plans and teacher certification programme is learning how to construct proper Google searches. For example, one freely available scheme of work consists of 15 lessons on teaching students how to search on Google.[4] In the first lessons, students learn how to pick the right search terms, and then put that into practice by trying to identify the authors of five different historical sources.[5–6]

The later lessons move on to the challenge of evaluating the credibility of sources. Students are given guidelines about what constitutes a reliable source. They then have to work out whether or not certain stories are true, like the 'Navy Ghost Blimp', and evaluate the trustworthiness of a series of articles on genetically modified food.[7] One of these lessons comes with a checklist for students to use to evaluate sources, featuring questions like 'Can you identify an author? A real name or an alias?', 'Is the author connected with an organization? If so, can you determine if it is a respected organization? Name the organization' and 'Does the author include a works cited or other links to provide additional resources or original source information? Identify one.'[8]

Google's teacher certification programme

The teacher certification programme is even more explicit about its aims. It tells teachers that 'we have access to every bit of info we need at all times. It is therefore no longer relevant to focus on teaching facts.'[9] Instead, teachers should focus on teaching students how to 'search smart'. This 'saves them valuable time and is a highly-demanded skill in the modern workplace.'[10]

A unit on 'teaching students online skills' states that the three 'search smart' basics are:

1. Choosing the right search terms
2. Understanding search results
3. Narrowing a search to get the best results

Google for Education: *Search Smart*, 2019

The unit provides more information about each of these, including how to use search modifiers and filters. These teacher guides also contain similar advice to the lesson plans: in order to evaluate the reliability of a webpage, it recommends that students ask themselves the following questions:

Who is the author(s) of the content? Do they have any special skills that qualify them to write on this topic?
Is the content trying to make you believe a particular point of view? Are there ideas or opinions that are missing?

Google for Education: *Boost Student Research Skills*, 2019

It also recommends that students apply the 'Rule of 3':

> An easy rule that can be applied when searching online is the 'Rule of 3'. Encourage all students to compare three sources of information before coming to a conclusion on any given topic.
>
> Ibid.

The Google for Education website features other lesson plans too, some written by Google and some by teachers. Few place any emphasis on what you might call 'traditional' classroom content: knowledge of literature, history, geography, chemistry, etc. In keeping with the idea that learning facts is irrelevant, few require students to learn any facts. More typical are lessons that work with knowledge students already have, without attempting to extend it.

One lesson plan is called 'How to eat a cupcake' and involves students writing step-by-step instructions about how to eat a cupcake using Google Docs.[11] Another lesson asks students to use Google Slides to create a presentation about themselves.[12] In another, students use social media to create a Twitter homepage for historical figures.[13]

If you think that teaching facts is irrelevant because students can easily look them up online, then these kinds of lessons make sense. What students really need to learn is how to use Google apps. The content they write about doesn't matter so much, because they can always look it up.

So, Google's claim is as follows: it's no longer relevant to learn facts because it is so easy to look them up, and students are better off learning a set of all-purpose tools or techniques that allow them to evaluate the quality of information once they have looked it up.

This is wrong, for the following three reasons:

1. We need facts in long-term memory because we use them to think, and without them our working memories would quickly get overwhelmed.

2. Even when we are using reliable online sources, we need facts in long-term memory to be able to look something up and make sense of what we find.

3. When we do encounter unreliable online sources, relying on generic evaluation skills will not help us to identify them.

Let's explore each of these in turn.

We need facts to think

The main reason why we still need to know facts is that long-term memory is not a minor or a separate part of human cognition. Instead, it is an extremely powerful part of human cognition, and one that is integrated with all of our mental processes.

> Long-term memory is now viewed as the central, dominant structure of human cognition. Everything we see, hear, and think about is critically dependent on and influenced by our long-term memory.
>
> Kirschner P. A., et al., 2006

In Chapter 1, we saw how the knowledge we have in long-term memory allowed us to interpret the word 'bank' in two very different ways. This type of knowledge is vital. We can't outsource it to the Internet. We are using it all the time, even when we don't think we are, in order to make sense of the world.

Some of the crucial experiments in this area were carried out in the 1970s by Herbert Simon and William Chase on chess players. They wanted to know how expert chess players were so good and how they could make brilliant moves after studying a board for just a few seconds. Their research has become a cognitive science classic. I've written about it in my two previous books, and do so again here because it is so significant and has many important implications.

Expert memory – a case study of chess players

Simon and Chase's first experiments show the power of the best chess players' memories. When grandmaster chess players were shown a chessboard for a few seconds, they were able to reproduce the 25 pieces on the board from memory with almost no errors. When given the same task, less-expert players and novices could only recall 8–12 pieces accurately. At first glance, this seems to suggest something about the superior working memory of chess grandmasters.[14]

However, Simon and Chase went on to repeat the experiment, but with one crucial difference. This time, they used the same number of chess pieces, but they placed them at random on the board rather than copying positions from an actual game. In this experiment, the novices and the grand masters all performed equally poorly and could only remember three or four pieces on average.[15]

The implication of this experiment is that we think by using our long-term memories. These expert chess players have memorized the typical patterns of thousands of chess games. When they see a chess end game and rapidly decide what move to make, they can do so because they can compare the game state to all the board positions they have stored in long-term memory. They aren't reasoning; they're recalling. Or rather, their ability to reason is bound up with recall.

And fascinatingly, even a small change in the structure of the problem significantly weakens their ability because the experts were no better than novices at remembering a random set of pieces.

This is a sign that we need subject-specific information in long-term memory to become expert. There aren't general strategies we can learn that make us expert across different subjects.

The importance of memory can be seen in many other fields. Reading, which we often assume to be an all-purpose general skill, is dependent on memory. Dan Willingham, the cognitive scientist, provides the following example of a sentence that has no difficult vocabulary, but that many native English speakers still find tricky to understand.

> I believed him when he said he had a lake house, until he said it's only forty feet from the water at high tide.
>
> Willingham, D. T., 2009, p.24

I've presented this sentence to hundreds of people at training sessions, and it is fascinating to watch their reactions. Some stare at it, baffled, and when asked to explain what it means make wild guesses about underwater houses and the challenges of building on marshy land. Other people understand the sentence easily and wonder why I am insulting their intelligence with such a trivial sentence. The crucial piece of information needed to make sense of this sentence is that lakes don't have appreciable tides.

Once you know this, not only does the sentence make sense, but you can make some more sophisticated inferences. Indeed, if you did know that lakes don't have appreciable tides, your mind may have moved on to trying out some tentative inferences about the character of the man who says he has a lake house: that he might be quite boastful, that he is materialistic, that his friends perhaps see through his boasts and mock him. None of this 'higher-order' thinking is possible without a quite basic bit of knowledge.

Another example from Willingham is the following:

> **This brain scan is fuzzy. Probably, the patient was wearing makeup.**
>
> Amplify, Center for Early Reading, 2018, p.13

The key two facts you need to make sense of that sentence are that brain scans use magnets and that makeup contains trace elements of metal, which interfere with the magnets.

As well as showing how important facts are, these sentences also show how you cannot rely on looking them up. With both sentences, if you don't know what each sentence means, it's also hard to work out what to look up to make sense of it.

But even with sentences where it is more obvious what to look up, such as sentences with one word you don't understand, an online search is still not a great strategy. Imagine attempting to read a book where you had to look up the meaning of a word every sentence: even with a fast Internet connection, reading would become slow and tedious.[16] Every time you look something up, you rely on limited working memory. The more you have to look up, the less space you have to notice other features of the text you are reading or problem you are solving.

But there are also further reasons why relying on the Internet for facts is flawed. Let's look at these now.

We need facts in order to 'look it up'

Internet misinformation is a real problem, and one we will explore more later in this chapter. However, before we do so, let's consider all the useful and reliable online sources that exist. If we direct students straight to an online dictionary or encyclopedia that we know is reliable, surely that's fine?

It isn't, because the ability to look up information requires a baseline of information. This is true of online sources, and also of print reference sources. In Chapter 1, I shared the anecdote of a student who used a thesaurus to replace the word 'good' and created the sentence, 'I am a congenial footballer'. A similar scenario is the subject of a 1987 paper by George Miller and Patricia Gildea. They gave 8-year-olds a target word and a traditional paper dictionary, and then asked them to look the word up and write a sentence using it. They got back sentences like 'Mrs Morrow stimulated the soup' and 'Our family erodes a lot'.[17]

How did this happen? The authors explain:

> In order to understand what the children did, you have to read carefully the same dictionary definition the child read. The child who looked up stimulate found stir up amongst the definitions ... A fifth grader looked up the unfamiliar word erode, found the familiar phrases eat out and eat away in the definition and thought of the sentence 'our family eats out a lot'. She then substituted erode for eats out.
>
> Miller, G. A. and Gildea, P. M., 1987

Looking up new words is a 'high-level cognitive task' which easily overwhelms limited working memory capacity. Children cast around for ways to simplify it and in doing so produce distorted sentences. As the paper concludes, 'for the average child in the elementary grades it is likely to compound interruption with misunderstood information.'[18] Students end up with no idea what the word means, or with the wrong idea.

This brings us to an important caveat regarding the use of all reference sources, whatever their format. When you know something about the topic you are researching, it becomes easier to construct a useful search, and easier to interpret the information you find. The paradox is that reference sources are most useful to people who know something about the topic they are looking up, and less useful to those who know nothing about it. This is why many adults frequently do find reference sources useful.

However, when adults think about how valuable reference sources are for them, it's possible that they don't realize why they can use them so successfully. When adults think about looking something up online or in a dictionary, they think of the mechanics of constructing the search or knowing the alphabetical principle. They forget about all the specific content knowledge needed to know what to search for and how to interpret the results.

The reason they forget this is that this type of knowledge is so fluent and so well-understood that they can assume it is innate and universal. This type of error is known as expertise-induced blindness: when experts forget what it was like to be a novice and forget about the knowledge they depend on in order to be expert.[19]

In Miller and Gildea's experiment, the children could use the dictionary correctly to *find* the word they were looking for. They understood the alphabetic principle and could apply it. What this study shows, is that gaining meaning from a dictionary requires more than just the alphabetic principle. Similarly, while it is useful to know that in Google, putting quote marks around a phrase lets you search for that precise phrase, or that adding a minus sign before a word lets you eliminate that word, these techniques alone are not what allow us to create meaning from an Internet search.

Even high-quality and reliable reference sources are not, on their own, enough. And, as we are all too aware, many online reference sources are not high-quality and reliable. Let's consider the problem of Internet misinformation next.

We need facts to make sense of lies

As we've just seen, knowing the alphabetic principle used in dictionaries is similar to knowing how to construct a Google search. Both are useful technical pieces of information, even if on their own they are not enough to guarantee you can find the source you need and extract meaning from it.

However, there is one important difference between the way we search print and online reference sources. With print reference sources, we go directly to the dictionary or encyclopedia itself, and the reliability of what we find therefore depends on the reliability of the source itself. But online, often we start not with the actual reference source, but with a search of the entire world wide web.

The advantage of this is that you have access to many different sources; the disadvantage is that you have no idea how reliable those sources are. Google's solution is for students to be taught critical thinking skills and search skills that will let them distinguish between reliable and unreliable sources. But these kinds of skills are not generic; they are tied up with specific content knowledge.

The Pacific Northwest Tree Octopus is a famous hoax website created in the 1990s. A fascinating study on this Internet hoax sheds some interesting light on this issue. It is an extremely small study on just 25 students, but it illustrates some broader themes that have been found in larger-scale research.

The Pacific Northwest Tree Octopus

The hoax website contains detailed and often amusing descriptions of an entirely fictitious creature.[20–21] In 2007, researchers at the University of Connecticut asked 25 seventh grade students to evaluate the reliability of the website.[22] All of them said the tree octopus was real, and 24 of them said that the website was 'very credible'. Even after the researchers told them the site was false, the students struggled to believe them. And as if that were not all bad enough, these 25 students had been specially selected as their school's 'most proficient online readers'.

It's unlikely that Google's search skills checklist would have helped these students identify the hoax. The checklist asks students:

- 'Can you identify an author? A real name or an alias?' The author of the Tree Octopus hoax is clearly stated at the bottom of each page – Lyle Zapato.

- 'Is the author connected with an organization? If so, can you determine if it is a respected organization? Name the organization.' It's associated with the 'Kelvinic University branch of the Wild Haggis Conservation Society'.

- 'Does the author include a works cited or other links to provide additional resources or original source information? Identify one.' The website has a whole list of links to other resources and sources. It includes links to reputable websites and makes it seem as though those websites agree with it.

Ultimately, adults can identify that this website is a hoax not because they employ the Google checklist or any other 'critical thinking checklist', but because they know about octopuses. They know that octopuses are not found in trees. They also know that the 'Kelvinic University branch of the Wild Haggis Conservation Society' sounds a bit odd.

Children fall for this hoax because they lack this knowledge. In the absence of this knowledge, getting students to 'question more' is not going to make a difference.

Larger-scale research shows similar findings. The international PISA assessment of 15-year-olds includes questions about the reliability of webpages. One question, taken by 25,000 15-year-olds in 19 different countries, asked students to explain whether a sensationalist web news article on the smell of pizza was 'a suitable source for you to refer to in a school science assignment about smell?'[23] Only 25% of the students responded adequately, a figure that was the same for other similar questions. One student said the text was reliable because 'it shows us heaps of stats to include in an assignment', another sign of how surface features can be misleading.[24]

The researchers concluded that:

> Most 15-year-olds students do not know how to begin evaluating material they encounter on the internet. There is ample evidence that a majority of students consider it first in terms of relevance or interest, rather than looking at the reliability of its source.
>
> Lumley, T. and Mendelovits, J., 2012, p.9

Of course, this does not prove that absence of knowledge was the problem. But it does suggest that teaching students how to reliably assess the quality of online sources is trickier than we might first have thought.

One other important difference between online and print reference sources is interactivity. Print sources are inert and do not react or change based on the way an individual uses them. Online sources, however, are interactive.

This can be enormously positive, as we saw in the previous chapter, with adaptive learning systems designed to locate and correct errors in understanding. However, it can also be negative. Many online sources are designed not to correct errors in understanding but often to reinforce them. Websites like YouTube and Facebook often recommend similar content to what you have previously liked in the past. In the case of YouTube, it's been alleged that their algorithms are set up to recommend progressively more sensationalist or even misleading content to try and hook you into the website.[25]

This makes the disadvantages of unguided learning from online sources even greater than the disadvantages of unguided learning from print reference sources. If a student gets the wrong idea about the meaning of the word 'erode', the dictionary isn't going to suddenly bombard them with half a dozen sentences that all reinforce that misunderstanding. But if they get the wrong idea about whether the earth is round or not, then YouTube may well bombard them with a lot of videos that reinforce their misunderstanding. Indeed, the recent resurgence of belief in a flat earth has been partly attributed to YouTube's algorithms promoting such videos.[26]

So, not only is it not possible to outsource knowledge to the Internet, but it is also not possible to rely on abstract critical thinking skills to evaluate the credibility of the knowledge we find there. It's also potentially risky given the way some online resources shape themselves to fit your misconceptions.

Of course, knowing how to search the Internet effectively is a valuable life skill. But as we saw in the previous chapter, you don't get better at learning independently by learning independently. The same is true of Internet searches: you don't get better at searching the Internet by searching the Internet. Currently, Google's advice is that students can find the content they need on the Internet. But we could just provide students with well-designed, pre-selected content instead. Paradoxically, in the long run, this will make them better at Internet searches, because they'll know what they are looking for.

Digital literacy is a vital and complex skill. Evaluating the reliability of online sources ultimately means evaluating competing truth claims, something that has consumed the minds of some of the world's greatest philosophers. It's trivializing this skill to assume that it can be taught through lessons on identifying the author of a source.

As E. D. Hirsch says, 'to give all children a chance to take advantage of the new technology means not only seeing to it that they have access to the technology but also ensuring that they possess the knowledge necessary for them to make effective use of it.'[27]

Technology can help in two more promising ways. First, we can use technology to create coherent and memorable content. Second, we can use technology to enhance memorization, not replace it. Let's explore each of these now.

Creating memorable content

Instead of relying on students finding out what they need to know from the Internet, we should think about how we can give them information that is not just reliable, but that has also been designed for learning.

Principles of multimedia learning

To understand more about the best way of presenting content, and how technology can help, we need to turn to the work of Richard Mayer. Together with his colleagues, he has developed about 30 principles of multimedia learning which provide a powerful guide to creating memorable learning content.[28–29] Let's explore three of them in detail:

1. The multimedia principle

2. The split-attention effect

3. The redundancy effect

The multimedia principle

One of the most fundamental is the multimedia principle, which is that presenting text and images together can enhance learning.[30] This is because our limited working memories have two channels, one verbal and one visual. So presenting verbal and visual information uses the full capacity of our working memory, and allows us to build more sophisticated mental representations of the concept we are trying to learn. When we see words and images together, we work to connect the two, a form of active mental processing that helps build understanding.

Here is an example from one of Mayer's experiments. One group of students were given the following explanation of a bicycle pump.[31]

How a Bicycle Pump Works

"As the rod is pulled out, air passes through the piston and fills the area between the piston and the outlet valve. As the rod is pushed in, the inlet valve closes and the piston forces air through the outlet valve."

Text-only explanation of how a bicycle pump works.[32]

Another group were given the following explanation.

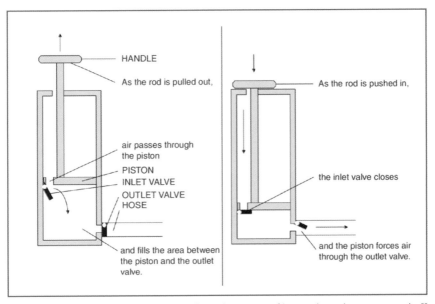

Text and image combined explanation of how a bicycle pump works.[33]

Both groups were then given a test to see not just if they had remembered the details of the pump, but if they could transfer their understanding to different situations; the second group did better than the first. This finding has been replicated in many other studies.[34]

The split-attention effect

Some other important principles qualify and develop the multimedia principle and give more detail on how to combine text and images. The split-attention effect shows that closely integrating text and images leads to better learning than providing the text and image separately.

Here's an example taken from an experiment by the academics Paul Chandler and John Sweller.[35] One group of trade apprentices received the following instructional material, consisting of an image and separate text instructions.

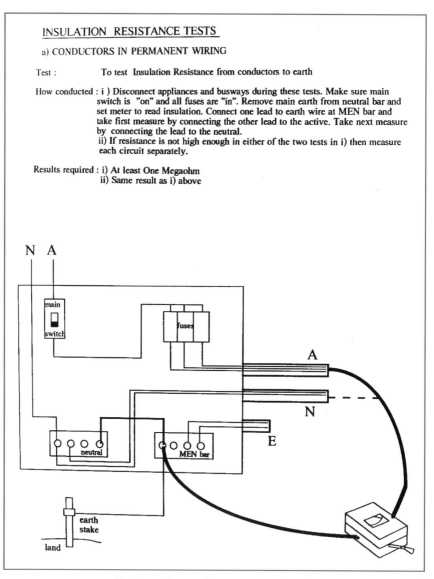

<u>INSULATION RESISTANCE TESTS</u>

a) CONDUCTORS IN PERMANENT WIRING

Test :   To test Insulation Resistance from conductors to earth

How conducted : i) Disconnect appliances and busways during these tests. Make sure main switch is "on" and all fuses are "in". Remove main earth from neutral bar and set meter to read insulation. Connect one lead to earth wire at MEN bar and take first measure by connecting the other lead to the active. Take next measure by connecting the lead to the neutral.
ii) If resistance is not high enough in either of the two tests in i) then measure each circuit separately.

Results required : i) At least One Megaohm
ii) Same result as i) above

Text and image kept separate insulation resistance tests.[36]

The second group received the same information, but the text was integrated with the image.

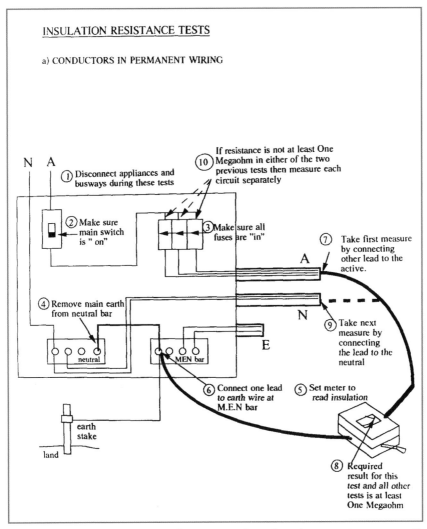

Text and image combined insulation resistance tests.[37]

The second group did better on both the written and practical tests that followed. Sweller and Chandler suggest that the reason for this is that the second group could devote all their attention to understanding the learning material. The first group had to spend more mental effort on a task that was unrelated to learning.

The redundancy effect

Another important principle that's particularly relevant to lectures and videos is the redundancy effect, which offers guidance on the way spoken word is presented.[38] Consider the resource about the bike pump which contains text and images. If a teacher were to give that resource to a class, how should they present it? Would it help to read out the text to the class, to make sure they were paying attention? The research says no. If learners have to deal with the same written and spoken words at once, they spend working memory resources coordinating the written and spoken words, meaning less working memory is available for learning.

Applying Mayer's multimedia learning principles

These are just three of about 30 multimedia learning principles. Others give advice on how important information is signalled to the learner, how it can help to progressively reveal content rather than present it all at once, and how it's important for all learning materials to exclude material that's not relevant to the learning objective.[39–41] And the 'expertise-reversal effect' shows that as students gain knowledge and understanding in an area, they can benefit from less-structured and scaffolded instructional materials.

These principles don't depend on certain technologies: Mayer is clear that they can be used in the design of worksheets, textbooks, digital slide presentations, videos and many other formats.[42] However, many of the principles do lend themselves well to newer technology. It's easy to combine images, texts and cues together in a digital presentation or a video, and easy to reveal information in progressive stages too.

Still, while digital media might make using such principles easy, they don't prevent misuse. Mayer's principles are incredibly powerful, but they are also quite complex and many traditional and digital learning materials violate them in one way or another. Modern technology makes it easy to integrate images and words in presentations, but it also makes it easy for teachers or lecturers to read out the words on a slide, violating the redundancy principle.

Similarly, while many presentations contain images, often these images are chosen for decorative purposes, and they can end up confusing or distracting learners. In the lesson on how bicycle tyre pumps work, Mayer recommends not including a photo or a video of a person riding a bicycle, as that is not relevant to the learning objective. Instead, he recommends 'using only highly relevant, instructional illustrations and even pointing out in the text what to look for in the illustrations.'[43]

Creating learning materials which fulfil these multimedia learning principles is not going to be easy, and nor will it happen by chance. Fortunately, we can learn from examples of content that has been specifically designed in accordance with these principles. In 2014, two academics, Barbara Oakley and Terrence Sejnowski, launched an online course that was deliberately designed with these principles in mind. Appropriately enough, the subject of their course was learning how to learn. The course has gone on to be one of the most popular Massive Open Online Courses (MOOCs) in the world. While the majority of the students enrolling are in the 25–34 age bracket, school-age students have enrolled too, and the creators have followed up with a book and course designed for younger learners.[44]

In 2019, they wrote a paper explaining how they'd applied Mayer's principles of multimedia learning to the creation of their course. Watching the videos from the course and reading the paper gives an insight into how these principles can be applied. For example, Oakley and Sejnowksi particularly focus on the learning benefits of green screen, as illustrated in the following image.

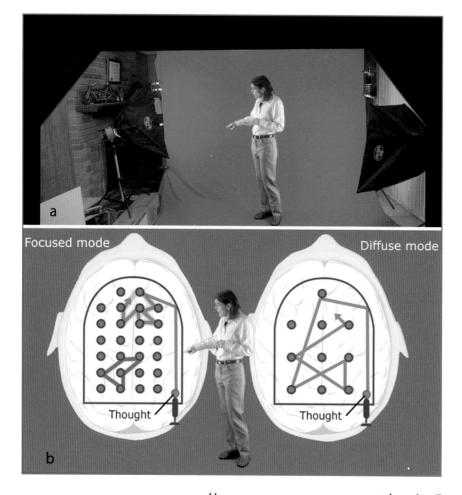

How a green screen can support learning.[45]

Green screen allows a video of the instructor to be inserted into the learning materials and for everything irrelevant to learning to be cropped out, reducing the extraneous load on working memory. You can also see that the images in this presentation have been chosen carefully to demonstrate the precise point the instructors want to make. They aren't decorative, easy-to-obtain clip art.

The result of all this is an engaging and extremely popular online course that embodies the principles it teaches. It's clear from watching these videos that not all content is created equal. Even reliable online information may not have been optimized for learning. In order to make sure students get the best learning materials, we have to create them, give them to students, and not rely on them stumbling upon them online by chance.

Oakley and Sejnowski's course doesn't only rely on well-designed content and explanations. In common with many other online courses, it provides frequent end-of-unit quizzes and in-video questions that let students check their understanding. Online quizzes like these have many benefits which we will explore in more detail in the next chapter. What we can see from this chapter is that instead of expecting technology to eliminate the need to build memories, we should instead use technology to make it easier for us to build memories.

The jobs of the future

Before we look in more detail at quizzes, however, let's deal with one more frequent objection to the idea that we need to know things. This is that, while we may need to memorize facts now, in the future rapid improvements in technology really will make memory obsolete and reduce the need for us to acquire complex skills. Perhaps learning a lot of foreign vocabulary is valuable now, but before long machine translation will improve to such an extent that we'll have *Star Trek*-style language earpieces. Perhaps learning how to map-read is valuable now, but before long we'll wear augmented reality headsets that will direct us to wherever we need to go.

It is true that computers are making rapid improvements in many areas, and we can expect this improvement to have an impact on jobs and the economy. However, while we can continue to expect technology to change the economy, this is not going to have the same impact on education for three reasons.

The first is that school education is concerned with more fundamental skills and knowledge that are less likely to be totally upended by technological changes. We can imagine a world in which self-driving cars mean less economic demand for driving instructors, but it is harder to imagine a world with less economic demand for people who can read, write and do basic mathematics. It is more likely that these will remain a prerequisite for many jobs in the future, even jobs that haven't been invented yet.

Second, many skills which are economically valuable depend on skills and knowledge which are not. Take mathematics: it used to be possible to get a job as a human computer, but technology has eliminated them, and no one is going to employ you simply because you know your times tables. However, you need to learn your times tables in order to master the more complex mathematics that employers do want. In order to acquire skills computers don't have, you may have to work through the ones they do.

The same is true of developing creativity: it's often said that in a world where technology is so good at recall, schools should teach creativity.[46] But creativity isn't a general skill.[47] Creative solutions aren't developed in a vacuum; new ideas tend to be developed by combinations of well-understood old ideas. In his history of scientific discovery, *Where Good Ideas Come From*, Steven Johnson shows how many transformative inventions are 'more bricolage than breakthrough' and gives several examples of how this works.[48] For instance, Johannes Gutenberg developed his printing press using his skills as a goldsmith and his knowledge of how wine presses worked. He succeeded not by 'conceiving an entirely new technology from scratch, but instead [by] borrowing a mature technology from an entirely different field, and putting it to work to solve an unrelated problem.'[49]

The third reason is that schools are not solely concerned with preparing students for the world of work. Schools are also preparing students to be successful adults and citizens.[50] So we shouldn't solely evaluate knowledge and skills in terms of their economic value. Indeed, historically, this has always been the case: we teach literature not because it has direct economic benefits, but because it helps students understand the world. Nor do we think that the aim of studying literature is for students to be 'better' at analysing it than a computer programme. Such an idea barely makes sense.

Given that we have never based our curriculum choices solely on economic value, we don't have to start to do so now.

- Suppose machine translation does result in more accurate and speedy translations that reduce the economic value of learning a foreign language. We might still choose to teach foreign languages on the grounds that they help students understand different cultures.

- Cameras have taken more accurate photos than human drawings for decades, but learning how to draw helps us to perceive the world in a different way.

- Online encyclopedias and maps can store more detailed and more accurate historical timelines and geographical maps than we can in our brains. But having a framework of world history and geography in our memories helps us make sense of new events.

We should evaluate what we teach in school based on the value it can give our students, not on whether we think it will let our students outperform technology.

For an analogy, let's consider physical machines like cars. The engine in a car turns fuel into energy, and modern engines have become more and more efficient at doing so. Humans also turn fuel, in the form of food, into energy, and are not as efficient at doing so as some of the most modern engines.[51-52] And of course, these engines are much more powerful and can propel cars in excess of 100 mph, far faster than any human capacity. These technological triumphs are great, and they are good for humans because they provide us with all the benefits of modern travel. The invention of cars and other forms of mechanical power also transformed the economy, reducing the economic need for manual labour.

So, machines are better at converting fuel into energy than humans, and the economic demand for human physical labour has declined as a result. But this doesn't mean we no longer need to eat, or worry about being physically healthy. Our fuel-to-energy conversion may not be that powerful or efficient, but of course we still need to eat because we have to eat to stay alive, and being physically healthy is part of leading a good life too.

Just as most people see eating as being about more than just fuel, memorizing facts is more than just something functional. We need facts in long-term memory in order to be able to think and make sense of the world around us. We can use technology to make memorization as fun as possible, we can use technology to make it as efficient as possible, but we cannot use technology to eliminate memory – unless we want to eliminate something that makes us human.

Summary

 We can't rely on search engines for knowledge

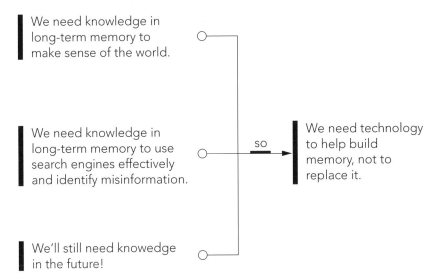

We need knowledge in long-term memory to make sense of the world.

We need knowledge in long-term memory to use search engines effectively and identify misinformation.

so

We need technology to help build memory, not to replace it.

We'll still need knowedge in the future!

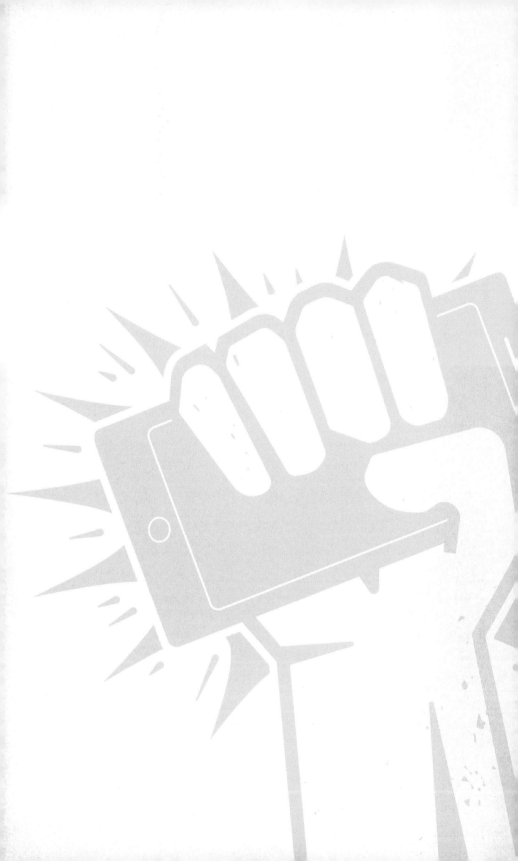

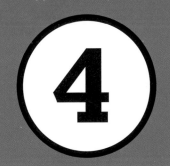

HOW CAN WE USE TECHNOLOGY TO MAKE LEARNING ACTIVE?

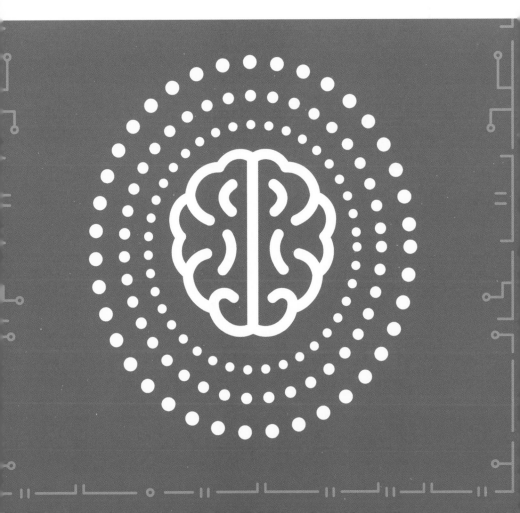

Different types of activity

In Chapter 1, we saw how the research into the science of learning showed that students need to be mentally engaged in order to learn. Some traditional teaching methods, like lectures, may make it easy for students to switch off and learn little. However, other methods, which claim to be active, have their own drawbacks. Complex tasks can overwhelm working memory. And some tasks define active learning very narrowly, in terms of the physical activity involved, rather than thinking more deeply about the cognitive activity that is needed for learning.

One of the great promises of technology is that it makes it easy to provide active and interactive instruction. But active learning, like personalized learning, is another phrase that gets defined in different ways. In this chapter I'll look at two particular approaches which often get classed as being active: projects and quizzes. I'll then consider different ways that we can teach complex skills, and provide a framework for thinking about the relationship between knowledge and skills.

Projects

The promise of project-based learning is that it lets students carry out more authentic projects that have more in common with the types of problems they will face in the real world. For example, instead of doing sentence drills and practising mathematics questions, students could carry out a project to evaluate the frequency and type of traffic around their school. By collecting the data and writing the project up, they will be learning about mathematics and English in a far richer context.

Project-based learning is not a new idea, but many technology companies have given it a new lease of life. In particular, both Microsoft and Apple recommend it as an approach to learning. In the previous chapter, we saw that Google's Chromebook has become the device of choice in many classrooms, but Microsoft and Apple still retain a strong presence in education systems around the world.[1] And like Google, they both provide professional development, sample lessons and recommended approaches to learning.

Microsoft have produced a professional development course for primary and secondary teachers about how to deliver problem-based learning. The course emphasizes the value of ill-defined and authentic tasks that use realistic contexts.

> If students are using data to solve a problem, they use actual data. For example, real scientific records of earthquakes, results of their own experiments, or first-person accounts of an historical event, not data developed by an educator or publisher for a lesson.
>
> Microsoft 21st Century Learning Design, *The Big Ideas*, 2019

Some of the specific projects Microsoft recommend giving students don't use much information technology: writing a persuasive letter to the head teacher about a change you would like to see in the school or designing a model house that will stay cool in the summer and hot in the winter.[2-3] Others, however, use Microsoft products to create real-world projects: one project requires students to develop a plan for combating loneliness among senior citizens by creating prototypes in Minecraft.[4] Another requires students to design a brochure about sustainable business practices for local businesses, using Photosynth, Movie Maker and Bing Maps.[5]

Apple's philosophy is captured in a guide they've produced about using the iPad in school called Everyone Can Create. It gives teachers ideas about projects they can use in the following curricular areas: mathematics; literacy and literature; history and social studies; science; and coding.[6]

At the start of the guide, they set out the reasoning behind their project ideas, using many of the phrases we've become familiar with already.

> We've developed the ideas to emphasize learning objectives that we know deepen student learning: real-world engagement, communication and creation, teamwork, critical thinking, and personalized learning.
>
> Apple, 2018, p.iii

Another part of the Apple website makes it even clearer, telling us that 'the best way to learn is by doing and making', and making it clear that the iPad is an ally in this work.[7]

Some of the projects recommended in the guide give us more detail about how this works in practice. For mathematics, Apple recommend a project called 'Equations Show', where students 'demonstrate how to solve equations with iMovie videos in the style of a cooking show. Use props to represent variables and numbers. Combine with other videos to create an equations cookbook.'[8] Another mathematics project 'Solve a Story', requires students to 'explain a mathematical theory through dramatization. Create an animatic [a series of images that play in sequence, like a storyboard] that builds in a math question or problem. Use the animatic to challenge others to provide solutions.'[9]

For science, a suggested project is 'Science Animations', where students use apps to 'explain a scientific concept with animations in Keynote. Export the presentation in movie format and open it in iMovie. Using iPad as a teleprompter, create a tutorial that explains the principle to others.'[10] To teach coding, the 'Silent Struggles and Successes' project is recommended. 'Share your emotions overcoming a coding hurdle through a silent film. Experiment with different ways to communicate the challenge visually, or use labels and stickers in Clips. Record your emotions in a selfie video, muting all sound and adding background music.'[11]

Silent films are also recommended for history, where the project 'Silent Communication' asks students to 'communicate news through a silent film. Create a newsreel in the style of the early days of silent film. Use a variety of shot types and add music.'[12] Finally, for literacy, in the 'Reading Reflection' project, students 'reflect on and analyse a story with video. Use Clips to record a reflection of the plot, style, characters and setting. Add Live Titles and posters as transitions.'[13]

The problem with all these activities is that they overload working memory. The very things that advocates love about projects – their real-world authenticity and complexity – are precisely the problem with them. Complex projects are just that: complex. The real world is not always a brilliant learning environment. The many elements of a typical authentic task can overwhelm working memory, meaning that even if students do manage to complete the project, they may not have learned anything from the process. The fundamental issue here is the one we've seen again and again: the mental activities we employ when solving a problem are different from the ones we use that develop the skill of solving that problem.[14] Let's look more closely at exactly why projects are so problematic.

We remember what we think about

In *Why Don't Students Like School*, cognitive scientist Dan Willingham sets out to provide teachers with useful, research-backed advice. In one chapter, he reveals what he considers to be 'the most general and useful idea that cognitive psychology can offer teachers.' It is this: 'review each lesson plan in terms of what the student is likely to think about.'[15] This is because we want students to remember what we teach them, and the way to remember something is to think about it. Or, to use another phrase of Willingham's, 'memory is the residue of thought.'[16]

At first sight, this might seem rather banal. Of course we should care about what students think about! Isn't that something that teachers do all the time? But while this advice may seem obvious, it has enormous implications for project-based learning. The problem with all kinds of projects – those that use technology, and those that don't – is that they involve so many different elements that it is hard to know what a student will pay attention to. Often, the important element you want students to focus on is obscured or unclear.

Willingham's examples of the kinds of activities to be wary about are similar to those promoted by Apple and Microsoft. In one lesson he observes, a social studies class go to the computer lab to prepare a PowerPoint presentation about the Spanish Civil War:

> The problem was that the students changed the assignment from 'learn about the Spanish Civil War' to 'learn esoteric features of PowerPoint'. There was still a lot of enthusiasm in the room, but it was directed towards using animations, integrating videos, finding unusual fonts, and so on.
>
> Willingham D. T., 2009, p.61

Of course it's useful to learn how PowerPoint and other popular computer programmes work. But in this lesson, the original aim was to learn about the Spanish Civil War, not about PowerPoint.

The specific projects recommended by Apple and Microsoft suffer from the same problem. If students are trying to make an iMovie video about equations that uses cooking utensils, how much time are they spending thinking about using iMovie and finding the cooking utensils, and how much time are they spending thinking about mathematics? If students are making a Minecraft world with the aim of combating senior-citizen loneliness, how much time are they thinking about creating the Minecraft world, and how much time are they thinking about the problem of loneliness?

If the sole claim were that these projects will help students get better at using iMovie and Minecraft, that would be fine. But the claim is that these lessons will help students learn mathematics, English, history, science and coding too. And, while learning how to use consumer software can be useful, it is clearly not all we should teach. The risk is that if project-based learning advocates make it seem as though you can learn every subject through the medium of iMovie, then students will end up learning iMovie in every class to the detriment of their study of mathematics, English, science and history.

Research into how these types of projects are used in schools does not offer reassurance. One Apple research project gave students in 114 underserved communities access to iPads, and monitored their impact.[17] The report noted that 'the percentage of teachers reporting daily classroom student use in their classroom [grew] from 31% in 2015 to 75% in 2017.'[18] It also found that students were spending most of their time looking up information online, creating presentations, and using 'newly available tools such as iMovie and GarageBand to create products that communicated their ideas.'[19] iMovie and GarageBand are two proprietary Apple products that allow users to create films and music.

Apple justify their projects by saying that they will help students to 'thrive in today's world and shape the future' and promote 'real-world engagement'.[20] And clearly, fluency with technology is an important part of surviving in the modern economy. But not all technological skills are equally valuable. Coding and data science are rare and valuable skills, which will help people to thrive in the modern economy, but it is not clear that using GarageBand has similar value. Cal Newport, the computer science professor, has a view on this. He criticizes the:

> ... absurdity of the now common idea that exposure to simplistic, consumer-facing products—especially in schools—somehow prepares people to succeed in a high-tech economy. Giving students iPads or allowing them to film homework assignments on YouTube prepares them for a high-tech economy about as much as playing with Hot Wheels would prepare them to thrive as auto mechanics.

> Newport, C., 2016, loc. 4390

For Newport, the skills that truly are valuable in the modern economy are best developed by intense and focussed concentration. The research on the limitations of working memory and the power of long-term memory suggests he is right.

More narrowly defined projects can work if teachers can be certain that students have the background knowledge and sub-skills needed to learn from them. In a mathematics class, if students have practised plotting a histogram extensively in different contexts, with practice data designed to show different possible distributions, then the next step could be to create a histogram of the heights of everyone in their class. These more limited projects have real value as the next step for students to take after mastering the necessary component parts. And the end goals – creating and interpreting a histogram – are skills that genuinely might be useful in later life, unlike many of the recommended projects we've seen which claim to involve real-world aims, but often just obscure important content with unnecessary distractions. It's unlikely that many students will ever be required to make a mathematics equation video out of cooking utensils in the real world.

And, of course, real-world projects can have extremely important non-academic purposes. A project to get students more involved with their local community by creating an allotment or café could be incredibly powerful. But Microsoft's recommended project here uses the virtual world of Minecraft, not the real world.

We should also be wary of assuming that a project has succeeded if a student manages to produce an interesting final product. Even if they do, they may not have learned anything from it, given the difference between using a skill and developing one. And those students who do create good projects may well have relied on background knowledge they have acquired from their families or from outside school. Again, we see the chicken-and-egg problem: projects require students to have knowledge without teaching them it, and the more projects are taught the less likely it is students will acquire the knowledge needed to succeed at them.

The testing effect: using technology to build memories

One effective method of active learning is simply to ask students a question about something they have learned. Simple quizzes encourage the type of cognitive activity that help build memories.

Still, while quizzing seems like a simple strategy, anything that involves testing is capable of being used and misused in many different ways. Many developed countries use big national assessments to determine how effective schools or teachers are, and these can distort wider educational goals.[21] 'Teaching to the test' can result in more of a focus on exam mark schemes than on the content of the curriculum. Multiple-choice questions can lead to gaming and guessing, and students can end up focussing too much on whether they got a question right or wrong, and not enough on why they got it right or wrong.

These problems can make it seem as though all assessment is bad. A typical criticism is that an excessive focus on test scores might measure attainment, but it won't help improve it. But, actually, testing can have a learning benefit. A great deal of research shows that the very act of retrieving something from long-term memory helps strengthen and consolidate that memory.[22] The challenge, therefore, is to avoid the distorting aspects of tests and to design and use them in the right way.

Many popular online mathematics and language learning programmes show how this can be done. Often, they consist of banks of thousands of questions of different types and difficulty, and the effort of recalling the right answers helps to consolidate understanding. One language learning app lets you add your own personal notes to tricky words to help you remember them; again, this is the type of mental activity that helps boost memory.[23]

One online mathematics programme integrates video instruction and questions. Students watch the videos, which take them through a series of worked examples, and then they immediately have to put into practice what they have watched by solving a new example of the same problem. Students immediately have to do something with the instruction they've received, making it more likely that they will understand it and start to build a long-term memory.[24]

Adding quizzes into lectures is also a simple way of making the lecture more interactive, as well as making it harder for students to mentally switch off. When students respond to quick questions throughout a lecture, it improves their understanding; some online platforms even make it easy to gather responses from all students in real-time.[25]

In order to build long-term memories, studying something once or twice is rarely enough. Digital quizzes make it easier to space out repetition of new content in the most effective way. Spaced repetition, which is also sometimes known as distributed practice, is one of the best-evidenced but least-used findings in education. It was first discovered by the memory researcher Herman Ebbinghaus in the late 19th Century, who also developed the idea of the 'forgetting curve'. Ebbinghaus's tests on his own memory showed that after learning something perfectly, he would start forgetting it almost immediately. After 9 hours, he forgot 60% of what he had learned, and after a month, 75%.[26]

His research also showed a way to interrupt this forgetting curve: by spacing out practice over time. He discovered that if he spaced out his study sessions over three days, he only needed half the amount of time to learn a list of syllables perfectly than if he crammed all his study into one session. The following graph illustrates the way the forgetting curve works, and how it can be interrupted by spaced practice.[27]

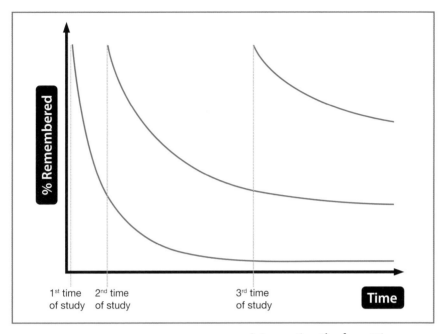

Interrupting the forgetting curve.

Ebbinghaus's findings have been replicated again and again in classroom situations and within different content areas.[28] In some ways, these findings are obvious: teachers are always telling their students not to cram revision into the night before an exam. However, in other ways, this research leads to some surprising conclusions that are not obvious. When we study a topic intensively in a short period of time, we can often display high levels of performance and feel confident that we have truly understood the material. But that feeling of confidence is misleading. In the words of Robert Bjork, a leading researcher in this area, performance is *not* the same as learning.[29] Spacing out practice may not give you the same fluency in the short-term, but it is far better in the long-term.

The spacing effect is not just relevant for exam revision: it has insights for the way we structure the curriculum itself. Despite this, however, it is not being used effectively. In 1988, one researcher described spaced learning as 'a case study in the failure to apply the results of psychological research.'[30] A 2007 review of the research suggested that little had changed in the interim.[31]

Traditionally, one of the practical challenges in implementing spaced repetition was finding the best moment to review the material, the sweet spot of 'desirable difficulty' where you have to struggle to recall something but haven't totally forgotten it.[32] Digital quizzing makes it easier to find this moment.

Many flashcards apps let you upload whatever questions you want, and they then determine how often to present each flashcard based on an algorithm that takes into account how often you've seen each card and got it right in the past.[33] Other websites are able to use information from testing to provide you with your own personal forgetting curve, based on how frequently you've studied:

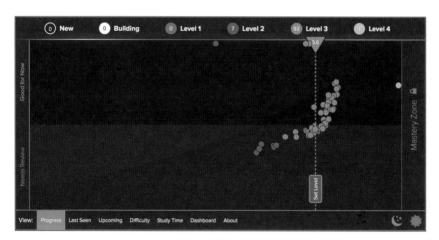

Cerego Memory Bank Progress Screen[34]

... each memory is represented as an individual orb, where the color and horizontal position shows the long-term retention built for that memory, and the height shows how active it is. As memories fade over time, the orbs drop in height and the learning engine will schedule them for review.

Harlow et al., 2016, p.22

The language learning app Duolingo has published research showing how it updates its learning algorithm based on findings from millions of students who use the app.[35] It shows how quizzes can add to the research in this area because it can aggregate data from millions of students and empirically see how long it takes to truly learn something. It can also tease out differences in different content: some words are harder to learn than others and require more repetitions. For example, it has found French-language learners find *visite* and *suis* easy to remember, but *fallait* and *ceci* much harder.[36]

If data from quizzes were collected in more subjects, we could start to see patterns and links between different content areas. We could find out if students who did a certain amount of practice on sentence drills in one year ended up writing better history or philosophy essays in later years, or if a certain amount of practice in algebra leads to better performance in chemistry. Some small-scale studies like this exist, but traditionally it has always been a challenge to carry out long-term studies of spaced repetition.[37] So using technology in this way offers the promise of both enhancing learning in the moment and offering insights about learning for future students.

Improving feedback

If you can only ever practise using complex problems, it's hard to zoom in on a particular weakness and work on it. Suppose a student struggles to understand how to use the apostrophe correctly. If you can only ever diagnose apostrophe problems and practise their correct use in the context of authentic extended pieces of writing, it will take a long time to work out exactly what a student's misunderstanding is. By contrast, a series of sentence drills spaced out over a series of lessons will be more effective at both diagnosing the problem and correcting it.

This diagnostic potential has been emphasized by K. Anders Ericsson, the world's foremost researcher in human expertise, who has studied the training and practice of experts in many different disciplines.[38] Often, just getting experience in an area is not sufficient to improve, as the following case study will show.

Improving a skill

In a 2005 paper, Ericsson and colleagues show that it is possible to play tennis regularly for 20 or 30 years and still not improve, because a typical game situation often doesn't provide great learning opportunities.

For example, if someone misses a backhand volley during a tennis game, there may be a long time before the same person gets another chance at that same type of shot. When the chance finally comes, they are not prepared and are likely to miss a similar shot again. In contrast, a tennis coach can give tennis players repeated opportunities to hit backhand volleys that are progressively more challenging and eventually integrated into representative match play.

Plant, E. A., et al., 2005

By breaking down a complex skill like this and focussing on one part of it, it's possible to quickly identify problems and to fix them. This doesn't only improve feedback for an individual, it also improves our understanding of learning in general.

This is the aim of the Diagnostic Questions website, which, at the time of writing, has hundreds of thousands of multiple-choice questions that have been answered by thousands of students. As well as selecting an answer, students can also provide their reasoning. For the following mathematics question, only 35% of students selected the correct answer, D, while an almost even split selected each wrong answer.[39]

Which number below is $\frac{3}{4}$ more than 0.5?

A	B	C	D
$\frac{4}{6}$	0.84	1.205	$\frac{5}{4}$

Multiple-choice question from an AQA test.

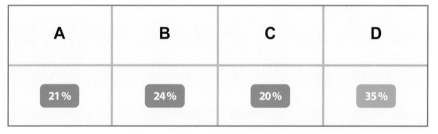

A	B	C	D
21%	24%	20%	35%

The percentage of students who selected each answer.

The reasoning of one student who chose the right answer reveals a solid understanding of fractions and decimals.

> ... because 3 over 4 is the same as 0.75 and 0.5 + 0.75 = 1.25. 5 quarters are the same as 1.25 because if you convert it into a mixed number then you have 1 and 1 quarter or 1 and 0.25
>
> Student explanation, cited in Barton, 2018

The explanations of students who chose the wrong answers are also revealing. One student who selected option A reasoned as follows:

$$\frac{3}{4} + \frac{1}{2} = \frac{4}{6}. \text{ Easy.}$$

Student explanation, cited in Barton, 2018

They've correctly turned 0.5 into a fraction, but then assumed, wrongly, that when adding fractions, you add the numerators (numbers on the top) and then add the denominators (number on the bottom).

However, some students who selected option A made a different error. They misread the question as 'Which number is below $\frac{3}{4}$ and more than 0.5?' and assumed they had to select a number between 0.5 and $\frac{3}{4}$.

$\frac{3}{4}$ is 0.75. $\frac{4}{6}$ is 0.6666666666 (so on) which is more than 0.5 however less than 0.75.

Student explanation, cited in Barton, 2018

It would be harder to spot these types of misconceptions within a more complex project. Diagnostic questions allow teachers to learn more about how their students think, and to identify the right activities that will help them improve.

Reducing cognitive load

Another advantage of this kind of testing is that by breaking down a complex skill into more manageable chunks, it reduces the load on working memory. Learning basic mathematics facts, for instance, is less overwhelming than trying to solve a complex mathematics problem. And, once you have memorized some basic facts, complex mathematics problems are easier to understand because they have the basic facts embedded within them.

Sometimes, simple and decontextualized quizzes are criticized for being atomized and divorced from real-world contexts. But isolating small aspects of a complex skill doesn't prevent students from gaining understanding; rather, it enables it by freeing up space in working memory to perceive the bigger picture.

Herbert Simon, John Anderson and Lynne Reder made this point in a paper in 2000 specifically on the educational applications of psychology. They argued that the insights from cognitive psychology showed us that it was possible to break down skills into their component parts and to practise them in isolation. They give the example of learning how to do multi-column addition. It's a good idea to practise this in isolation. You don't have to learn how to do multi-column addition through the real-world context of calculating income taxes, for example.[40]

In the same paper, Simon et al. emphasize the crucial role of practice in building competence. They criticize the pejorative phrase 'drill and kill' for suggesting that practice must be demotivating:

> The instructional task is not to "kill" motivation by demanding drill, but to find tasks that provide practice while at the same time sustaining interest.
>
> Anderson, J. R., et al., 2000

This is another area where technology can help, by making routine and regular practice fun and stimulating. One great example of this is an online times tables practice programme where students acquire a rock star avatar, and can upgrade their status to a 'rock hero' the more correct questions they answer.[41] They can also compete with students from their class and other schools. The same developers have created a similar programme for practising adding and subtracting facts.[42]

Breaking down complex tasks

Still, while breaking complex tasks down into smaller chunks is helpful, some wariness is understandable. The exact choice of how to break something down and in what ways is often not straightforward.

For mathematics, it can be quite obvious that fluency in basic mathematics facts is necessary, and it's also fairly obvious which facts are important. We *do* expect students to memorize the following:

×	1	2	3	4	5	6	7	8	9	10	11	12
1	1	2	3	4	5	6	7	8	9	10	11	12
2	2	4	6	8	10	12	14	16	18	20	22	24
3	3	6	9	12	15	18	21	24	27	30	33	36
4	4	8	12	16	20	24	28	32	36	40	44	48
5	5	10	15	20	25	30	35	40	45	50	55	60
6	6	12	18	24	30	36	42	48	54	60	66	72
7	7	14	21	28	35	42	49	56	63	70	77	84
8	8	16	24	32	40	48	56	64	72	80	88	96
9	9	18	27	36	45	54	63	72	81	90	99	108
10	10	20	30	40	50	60	70	80	90	100	110	120
11	11	22	33	44	55	66	77	88	99	110	121	132
12	12	24	36	48	60	72	84	96	108	120	132	144

But we *don't* expect students to memorize the following:

×	425	426	427	428	429	430	431	432	433	434	435	436
425	180625	181050	181475	181900	182325	182750	183175	183600	184025	184450	184875	185300
426	181050	181476	181902	182328	182754	183180	183606	184032	184458	184884	185310	185736
427	181475	181902	182329	182756	183183	183610	184037	184464	184891	185318	185745	186172
428	181900	182328	182756	183184	183612	184040	184468	184896	185324	185752	186180	186608
429	182325	182754	183183	183612	184041	184470	184899	185328	185757	186186	186615	187044
430	182750	183180	183610	184040	184470	184900	185330	185760	186190	186620	187050	187480
431	183175	183606	184037	184468	184899	185330	185761	186192	186623	187054	187485	187916
432	183600	184032	184464	184896	185328	185760	186192	186624	187056	187488	187920	188352
433	184025	184458	184891	185324	185757	186190	186623	187056	187489	187922	188355	188788
434	184450	184884	185318	185752	186186	186620	187054	187488	187922	188356	188790	189224
435	184875	185310	185745	186180	186615	187050	187485	187920	188355	188790	189225	189660
436	185300	185736	186172	186608	187044	187480	187916	188352	188788	189224	189660	190096

The 1–12 times tables are valuable because they recur again and again in more complex mathematics problems. Not all mathematics facts have the same value.

To teach a complex skill, we have to create what education professor Dylan Wiliam calls a 'model of progression', which is when we 'break down a long learning journey into a series of small steps'.[43] While the end goal is a complex skill, the small steps often involve learning facts and knowledge.

Facts and knowledge can be useful building blocks even when our end goal is to encourage a personal response to a literary text. I realized this when teaching *A Midsummer Night's Dream*. Throughout the play, the main four characters fall in and out of love with each other due to the actions of a powerful love potion. Students love the calamities and fights that ensue after the potion has done its work, but they also struggle to keep track of who is in love with whom at which point.

For a lot of the play, that doesn't necessarily impede their understanding. But at the end of the play, the love potion has been removed from three of the four characters, but not from one of them – Demetrius. As a result, while three of the four characters are in love with who they were at the start of the play, Demetrius is about to get married to a woman who, without the effects of the love potion, he'd loathe.

When I first taught this play, I wanted my students to discuss the implications of this. But they were so shaky about who was in love with whom at different moments that they didn't completely understand what had happened.

Later in my career, I worked on an English curriculum that was explicitly designed to give students a solid grounding in who loved whom and when. At the beginning of the unit, this looked almost absurdly trivial, requiring numerous simple and repetitive closed questions. But at the end of the play, this all began to pay dividends. Students realized spontaneously, without being told, that Demetrius was in love with a woman he had loathed.

Some students were fine with that, but others were outraged. Some felt it was fine to be deceived if it led to you being happy, but others felt that truth was more important than happiness. In short, they engaged in some quite sophisticated discussions about the value of truth, but it was all predicated on some basic and apparently trivial questions earlier in the unit. When students thoroughly understand something, it makes it easier for them to come up with spontaneous and original insights.

Breaking down writing

Writing provides another interesting case study of breaking down a complex skill. Writing can be taught as part of more complex cross-curricular projects, in which case it is hardly broken down at all. Students are just expected to write up reports about various different topics and, in doing so, learn how to write.

Or, writing can be broken down according to genre, with students studying the features of persuasive, analytical and creative writing, and then employing these features in their own writing.

Both these approaches are on display in Microsoft's recommended lessons: in one, students write a letter about their science project, and in another they identify the features of persuasive writing before writing their own persuasive letter.

Both these approaches were common when I trained to teach, but I grew frustrated with them because they provided so little time to address the technical flaws in my students' writing. In particular, I wanted to focus more on sentence structure, which isn't a trivial or pedantic concern, but one that goes to the heart of good writing. Many of my students wrote essays full of run-on sentences, which made it hard to understand their meaning.

Of course, I would feed back to students that they needed to use more full stops, but this was a reactive and piecemeal way of responding to something far more fundamental. And even when students did pay attention to this feedback, it would often just result in them adding full stops in the wrong place, and creating lots of sentence fragments instead.

My students didn't just need to be told to use more full stops. They needed to know *where* to put a full stop. And in order to know that, they needed to know what the subject of a sentence was, and what the main verb was.

Teaching verbs

However, in many ways this just created new difficulties about the best way to teach subjects and verbs. A lot of my students had learned that a verb was 'a doing word'. This can seem like a helpful definition for beginners. I'd give them sentences like the following:

> I run to the shops.

Armed with the definition 'a verb is a doing word', they would successfully identify that 'run' was the verb.

However, ultimately this definition caused more problems than it solved. Take this sentence:

> I went for a run to the shops.

Students would be equally confident that the verb in this sentence was 'run'. When I told them it was 'went', they would struggle to understand why. How can 'went' be a doing word? And how come run is a verb in one sentence, but not in another? Similarly, sentences like this one would prove tricky.

> I really like my gymnastics class.

Students would assume that gymnastics was the verb, because it involved action, instead of identifying 'like' as the verb.

Of course, other definitions of a verb are possible. But none of them seemed to help students to truly understand. It's experiences like these that make many teachers give up on explicit grammar instruction, and conclude that perhaps the understanding of correct sentence structure can only be 'picked up' through exposure to real writing.

However, there is another way of teaching the building blocks of writing. The Direct Instruction programmes I mentioned in Chapter 1 don't assume that students can pick up the correct rules of writing just by reading or writing real texts. But neither do they teach students through rules. Instead, they teach using examples, but carefully constructed examples that are designed to illustrate a general principle.

Expressive Writing, the Direct Instruction programme, doesn't tell students that verbs are doing words.[44] Instead, it gives them lots and lots of sentences where the verb is highlighted, and then it gives them more sentences where they have to identify the verb. They move on to writing their own sentences, paragraphs, and longer stories and articles. As well as this, the activities are all sequenced so that practice of the same concept is spaced out over time.

The choice and sequencing of examples is vital. Siegfried Engelmann, the designer of Expressive Writing and the successful DISTAR Direct Instruction programmes we saw in Chapter 1, explains this in a guide he has written. Suppose you give students the following set of sentences to help them understand what a verb is.

He *ran* home.

She *ate* an apple.

I *fell* out of the boat.

You *slept* like a baby.

Engelmann, S. and Colvin, G., 2006, p.37

In these examples, all the verbs are the second word in the sentence, and they are all past tense and irregular. The examples therefore don't illustrate all the features of verbs, and so can lead to students developing misconceptions. Suppose they then read this sentence.

> Every day, she *plays* football.

They might assume that 'day' is the verb, because it is the second word.

The trick is to devise a series of examples that prevent such misconceptions and encourage the right inference. Here is Engelmann's example of a better series of examples to teach what verbs are.

> The old man *shovels* snow.
>
> Her car *slid* down the hill.
>
> Kim *worked* very hard.
>
> Those horses *run* around the field.
>
> A flock of blackbirds *makes* a lot of noise in the morning.
>
> The winner of the race *set* a new record.
>
> I *rode* for 12 hours.
>
> Sandra *studies*.

Engelmann, S. and Colvin, G., 2006, p.39

Here, the verbs are not all past tense, and they don't always appear as the second word in the sentence. They encourage the right inference. This is different from learning from authentic contexts like novels or conversations, where we cannot be sure that examples will support the correct interpretation.

Something similar is true of the acquisition of vocabulary. We saw the experiments in the previous chapter that showed the difficulty of learning new words through definitions, for example, when a child confused 'erode' and 'eat out'. In a practical guide to teaching vocabulary, Isabel Beck recommends teaching new words through examples, but again, carefully constructing those examples to prevent misconceptions. Authentic texts that contain irony can be particularly misleading, as Beck shows. A student who tried to work out the meaning of the word 'dire' from the following text would probably get it completely wrong.

> Gregory had done all he could to complete the task. When Horace approached his cousin he could see that Gregory was exhausted. Smiling broadly, Horace said, "You know there are dire results for your attempt."

Beck, I. L., et al., 2013, p.6

Different models of progression

To sum up, for writing we've looked at three different models of progression: learning by doing, learning by rules, and learning by practising with carefully constructed examples. It's the latter that is most likely to succeed.

Learning by doing and learning by rules seem like they are total opposites. Hands-on projects seem progressive and modern; rules and definitions seem quite traditionalist and old-fashioned. But they have more similarities than you might think, because neither approach breaks down complex content in a way that makes it easy to understand.

And sometimes, these two apparently opposite approaches get combined. A number of Microsoft's recommended lesson plans feature complex real-world projects that are accompanied with rubrics that provide teachers with guidelines for assessing the projects. The rubrics consist of generic rules about how the project should have been accomplished which are quite similar to abstract rules and definitions. For example, the project about creating sustainable businesses says that an exemplary project will:

> Provide comprehensive insight, understanding, and useful tips for sustainability in your assigned aspect of business.
>
> Microsoft 21st Century Learning Design, *Anchor Lesson*, 2019

Whereas a project that is only proficient will:

> Provide a moderate amount of insight, understanding and useful tips for sustainability in your assigned aspect of business.
>
> Ibid.

These rubrics are supposed to be used not just for grading, but also to provide feedback for the students so that they can improve their work. But how helpful is it to tell a student that their work is 'moderate', and to improve they need to make it 'comprehensive'? As Dylan Wiliam points out, the types of language used on these rubrics are not that helpful.

> I remember talking to a middle school student who was looking at the feedback his teacher had given him on a science assignment. The teacher had written, "You need to be more systematic in planning your scientific inquiries." I asked the student what that meant to him, and he said, "I don't know. If I knew how to be more systematic, I would have been more systematic the first time." This kind of feedback is accurate—it is describing what needs to happen—but it is not helpful because the learner does not know how to use the feedback to improve. It is rather like telling an unsuccessful comedian to be funnier—accurate, but not particularly helpful, advice.
>
> Wiliam, D., 2011, p.120

Dan Willingham makes a similar point:

> If you remind a student to "look at an issue from multiple perspectives" often enough, he will learn that he ought to do so, but if he doesn't know much about an issue, he *can't* think about it from multiple perspectives.
>
> Willingham, D. T., 2007

In Chapter 7 we will look in even more detail at the problems with these kinds of rubrics and potential ways to replace them.

Pendulums or pathways?

We can sum up the central messages in this chapter with a couple of diagrams. Educators have often criticized some of the traditional methods of teaching, such as those that use lectures, rules and definitions, as not being active enough. And there is definitely some truth to this. However, learning by doing with real-world, hands-on projects is misguided too, because our limited working memories make it hard to learn from complex environments.

One response to this problem is to acknowledge both extremes are wrong and to call for more balance instead. That's exactly what Summit Learning do here:

> In education, there is often a tendency for the pendulum to swing in one direction or another. Teaching that exclusively focuses on rote memorization does not motivate students or necessarily lead to retention in long-term memory. At times, groups of educators have called for a complete departure from the teaching of Content Knowledge in favor of approaches that are more hands-on or have focused on skills acquisition without any intentional teaching of content. We have carefully studied the history of these pendulum swings, and in taking stock of the evidence at our disposal at this time, we have concluded that Summit Learning will adopt an approach that focuses on both the acquisition of Content Knowledge and the development of Cognitive Skills.
>
> Summit Learning, 2017, p.40

However, while this call for balance can seem sensible, it just ends up reinforcing an unhelpful distinction between knowledge and skills. The metaphor of the pendulum swing tells us everything we need to know. This view of knowledge and skills imagines them as two polar opposites and sees the challenge as being to get the pendulum at the right point between the two extremes.

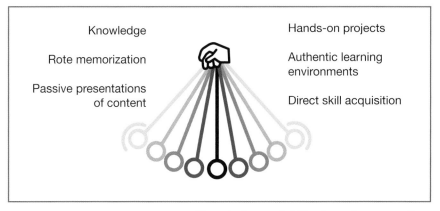

Knowledge and skills viewed as opposites.

The problem with calling for a balance between these two extremes is that they are both fundamentally flawed. Trying to strike a balance between the two often just ends up combining two ineffective methods: giving students a lecture or a factsheet before setting them off on a minimally guided project, or getting students to complete a complex real-world task which is then given feedback using an abstract rubric.

Indeed, the popular notion of 'flipped learning' falls into this trap of balance. Flipped learning generally involves students watching a video or reading a factsheet outside of class, so that the lesson can then be spent on independent projects.[45] The idea is that the video or factsheet can provide the knowledge, and then the project provides the skills. But ultimately, all of these activities are relatively unstructured and provide no guarantee that students will mentally engage with useful content.

A 2018 meta-review of 71 flipped-learning papers found the most commonly reported problems were students not engaging with or understanding the task they had to do before the class.[46]

The solution is not to find a halfway house between two ineffective methods. The solution is a completely different conception of education altogether. This conception of education should start with the complex skills we want students to acquire. After all, these are the final aims of education. If all students can do at the end of school is parrot some disconnected facts, we've failed. We want them to use their mathematics to solve the real problems they will face in life, to use language to communicate effectively, and to have insight into current affairs thanks to what they have learned in history and geography.

Once we've established the complex skills that are our aim, we then have to think about the best way of achieving those aims: the small steps on the long learning journey. And these smaller steps will look different from the end goal itself, as we break down the complex skill into the knowledge, sub-skills and examples that will allow students to develop it.

A better metaphor might therefore be knowledge as a pathway to skill. The pathway is not necessarily linear or straightforward: in order to learn, we need multiple representations of a concept, spaced over time. But the pathway metaphor helps us to see that it makes no sense to use phrases like 'a balance of knowledge and skills'. As the educationalist Heather Fearn says, this is like saying 'a balance of cake mixture and cake'.[47]

The pathway metaphor can also help us to identify more or less effective ways of achieving our end goals. Learning through examples is particularly effective. Short quizzes and spaced practice can help students consolidate long-term memories. And some knowledge is more useful than others. By contrast, learning through complex projects or rules and definitions is less effective. What follows is an image showing what a pathway towards the complex skill of writing might look like.

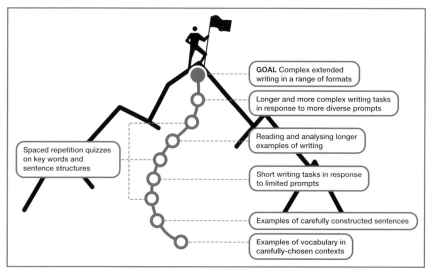

A pathway to the complex skill of writing.

The challenge for educators is to work out the most effective and efficient pathway to success for the different goals we want our students to achieve.

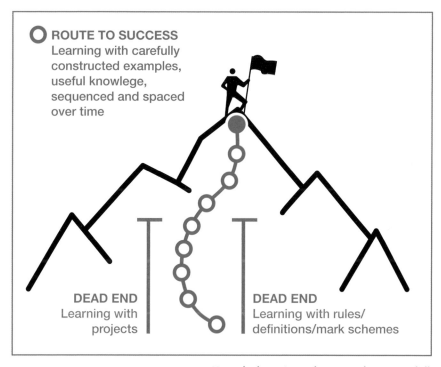

Knowledge viewed as a pathway to skill.

This isn't a new idea: back in 1969, Herbert Simon suggested that this kind of exploration and conquering of 'inner space' could be as exciting a challenge as the recent moon landings.

> The exploration of the moon is a great adventure. After the moon, there are objects still farther out in space. But man's inner space, his, mind, is less well known than the space of the planets. It is time we establish a national policy to explore this inner space systematically, with goals, timetables, and budgets. Will you think me whimsical or impractical if I propose that one of these goals be a world-champion chess-playing computer program by 1975; and another, an order-of-magnitude increase by 1980 in the speed with which a human being can learn a difficult school subject, such as a foreign language or arithmetic?
>
> Simon, H. A., 1969, p.52

In 1969, many would have dismissed the idea of a world-champion chess computer as absurd. But, while it took us longer than Simon anticipated, we have achieved that goal. The seemingly more mundane goal of increasing the speed of learning a school subject has not been achieved. And, as we saw in the last chapter, we seem less interested in developing human intelligence than in replacing it with artificial intelligence.

But if we want to focus technology on developing human intelligence, there are enormously exciting prospects. Learning apps are capable of aggregating millions of data points to work out the most effective ways of sequencing practice. We can test different ways of breaking down complex skills to work out which are the best. In subjects like mathematics, early reading and foreign language learning, where we already have a lot of research, this could lead to improvements. In other subjects where we have less research, it could lead to transformation.

However, these kinds of innovations will only be possible if we accept the limitations of our working memory, and the consequent value of breaking down complex skills into smaller parts. Unfortunately, a cavalier and wasteful attitude to human attention is central to much of modern technology. In the next chapter we will look at the problem of attention more closely.

Summary

In order to learn, our minds need to be active

Complex and authentic tasks seem like they will promote mental activity, but in fact they can overwhelm our limited working memories.

COMPLEX TASKS ARE THE END GOAL, NOT THE STEPS ON THE WAY.

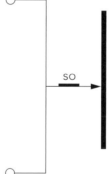

SO

We need digital quizzes that build up to a complex skill, making it easier for students to learn and helping us to learn the most effective ways of organising a curriculum.

Breaking complex tasks down into smaller chunks makes it easier for us to learn.

QUIZZES ARE A GREAT WAY TO LEARN BECAUSE THEY FORCE US TO BE MENTALLY ACTIVE BUT THEY DON'T OVERWHELM WORKING MEMORY.

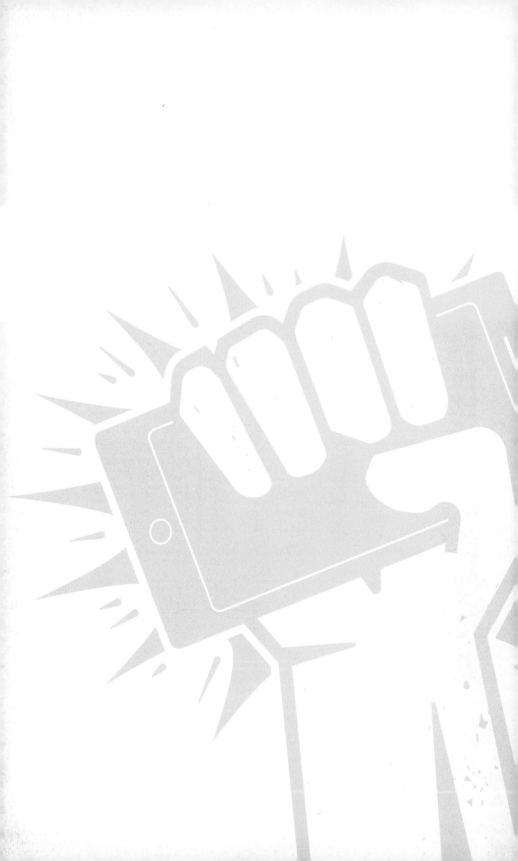

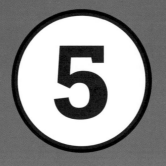

HOW SHOULD WE USE SMART DEVICES?

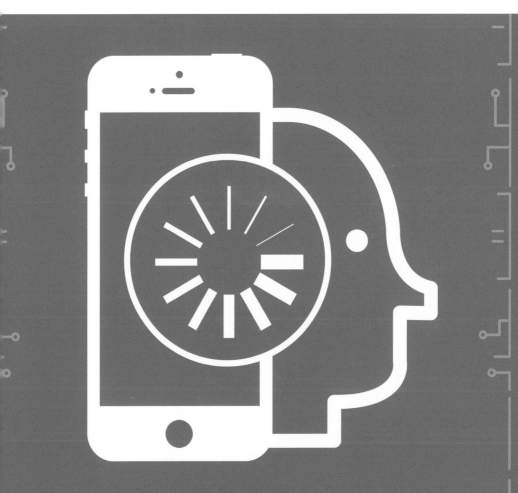

Computers, tablets and phones

So far, the various different technological approaches we've looked at have depended on students having easy access to connected devices. Often, it's assumed that getting connected computers, laptops, tablets or mobile devices into the hands of every learner is a prerequisite for learning. And some would go further and argue that connected devices are all that a student needs in order to learn.

The One Laptop Per Child (OLPC) programme was launched in 2005 with the aim of providing all students in developing countries with laptops, on the basis that this alone would be enough to educate them.[1] The founder of OLPC, Nicholas Negroponte, said that:

> One of the things people told me about technology, particularly about laptops in the beginning, "Nicholas, you can't give a kid a laptop that's connected and walk away." Well you know what, you can. You actually can. And we have found that kids in the remotest parts of the world, when given that connected [laptop] … not only teach themselves how to read and write, but most importantly, and this we found in Peru first, they teach their parents how to read and write.
>
> Nicholas Negroponte, quoted on *OLPC News*, 2010

Similar claims have been made by Sugata Mitra, an academic famous for his 'Hole in the Wall' experiments where he installed a computer in a kiosk in an Indian village and monitored the effects. Mitra developed a theory of 'Minimally Invasive Education' based on this, which similarly suggested that access to a computer connected to the Internet would allow students to learn computing skills 'and many other subjects as well'.[2]

> The MIE (Minimally Invasive Education) approach would involve exposing the learner to the learning environment without any instruction. In the case of computer literacy, the learner should be provided with a multimedia computer connected to the Internet.
>
> Mitra, S., 2010, p.19

OLPC did not manage to succeed at the scale it hoped for, but in some ways the market has fulfilled similar aims. The price of mainstream tablets has come down sharply, making them more and more accessible to schools and students across the world.[3] And the even more dramatic spread of mobile devices means that millions of students globally are connected to the Internet.[4–5]

Unfortunately, on its own, giving students connected devices achieves little. Bill Gates acknowledged as much when he said that 'just putting devices in classrooms has a really lousy record'.[6] While Negroponte may have claimed that students with laptops can teach themselves and their parents to read, evaluations of OLPC show it has made little difference to educational outcomes.[7] A 2017 meta-analysis of a variety of different technology access programmes, including some from OLPC, concluded that they did not 'measurably improve academic achievement'.[8]

The Hole in the Wall project has never been properly evaluated, but reviews have shown that many of the computers were vandalized shortly after installation, that students mostly used them to play games and watch movie clips, that no content was provided in Hindi (the language of the students) and that the computers were monopolized by older boys.[9–10]

Devices aren't neutral

Negroponte and Mitra's faith in the power of smart, connected devices may be unusual in its degree, but it is not that unusual in kind. It is part of a broader trend we have seen in the past few chapters which neglects thoughtful and well-designed content in favour of the apparently transformative power of new technologies and media.

This prioritizing of medium over content has its philosophical roots in the work of Marshall McLuhan, the media theorist who developed the idea that 'the medium is the message.'[11] This famous phrase has been interpreted in many different ways, but one extreme interpretation is to say that content doesn't matter. Certain media have certain styles or attitudes that transcend content:

> It doesn't matter if the networks show twenty hours a day of sadistic cowboys caving in people's teeth or twenty hours of Pablo Casals droning away on his cello in a pure-culture white Spanish drawing room. It doesn't matter about the content. The most profound effect of television – its real 'message', in McLuhan's terms – is the way it alters men's sensory patterns.
>
> Wolfe, T., 1967, p.18

This idea has become famous, and many of the popular, content-light approaches to education we've seen so far have perhaps been influenced by it, even if only indirectly.

We've also seen that these approaches don't work. Content does matter. Some of the early research on this was done in the 1970s by educational psychologist Richard E. Clark. Back then, television was the exciting new medium, and the hope was it could transform education and instruct students better than any traditional medium. Clark's 1983 meta-review showed that the educational benefits of TV were exaggerated, and concluded that:

> Consistent evidence is found for the generalization that there are no learning benefits to be gained from employing any specific medium to deliver instruction.
>
> Clark, R. E., 1983

And he came up with a metaphor to explain this idea which was the opposite of McLuhan's aphorism:

> Media are mere vehicles that deliver instruction but do not influence student achievement any more than the truck that delivers our groceries causes changes in our nutrition.
>
> Ibid.

Almost 40 years on, we can see that education is still unfortunately too keen on investing in shiny new trucks rather than healthy foods.

Clark's reminder of the importance of content is as important and necessary now as it was in the 1970s. However, his assumption that the medium is neutral may not be quite right. What if the 'medium is the message' idea does have some truth to it? But what if, far from this meaning we should be more enthusiastic about modern media in education, it means we should be *less* enthusiastic?

The extreme reading of 'the medium is the message' is clearly wrong. However, a subtler and more limited reading of it does have some truth. This reading would be that content clearly matters, but that the type of content that can be expressed through some media is different from others. Technological devices are not neutral carriers that can be loaded up with any type of content.[12] Rather, certain devices make certain types of messages and content easier to deliver, and therefore make such content more likely to be presented than others, as Neil Postman, the educationalist, explains:

> To take a simple example of what this means, consider the primitive technology of smoke signals. While I do not know exactly what content was once carried in the smoke signals of American Indians, I can safely guess that it did not include philosophical argument. Puffs of smoke are insufficiently complex to express ideas on the nature of existence, and even if they were not, a Cherokee philosopher would run short of either wood or blankets long before he reached his second axiom. You cannot use smoke to do philosophy. Its form excludes the content.
>
> Postman, N., 1985, pp.6–7

Of course, a book and a smoke signal are different. But even smaller and subtler differences between media have a big impact on the type of message that is communicated.

For example, it's possible to read the same political essay in many different formats. Reading it on a website browser accessed through a desktop computer is different from reading it on a mobile application, which is different again from reading it as part of a paper book. In *Words Onscreen*, Naomi Baron, a professor of linguistics, reviews the differences between reading in different formats, and emphasizes the trade-offs: 'when reading on a digital device with an Internet connection, you can check out a reference on the web—but you are also more likely to get distracted.'[13] And when authors know they are writing for a certain format, it can change the types of messages they communicate, in obvious and less obvious ways. For example, most authors will have a different style when they are communicating on social media than when they are writing books.

This is not to say that certain media are universally better or worse than others, simply that each has its own benefits and weaknesses. Different technologies are good for some purposes, and less good for others, and this is true even of powerful modern smart devices which are capable of fulfilling many different purposes. The same desktop computer can run an accounting programme, a drawing programme and a movie player, unlike older machines which were more specialized. In this strict technical sense, our modern devices are general-purpose.

However, sometimes this misleads us into thinking that because we can run any programme on our computers, that all programmes are equal and it's just up to us to choose what we want to do. This is not the case. Although all smart devices can run the same programme, some devices are designed to encourage the use of some programmes and not others. Both laptops and mobiles can run messaging programmes and word-processing programmes. But you generally don't see people on the street walking along with a laptop in front of them messaging their friend their location. And you don't see authors at their desks tapping out their latest novel on their mobile phone.

Later on, we will look more closely at the differences between desktops, laptops and mobile phones. But for now, we will spend some time looking at one important feature they have in common: their connectivity.

Connectivity and human attention

Being connected to the Internet means being connected to a vast and ever-changing array of information. However, while the information may be virtually limitless, our attention is not. One of the first people to understand the importance of this imbalance between information and attention was Herbert Simon. He observed that in a world where information is free, what will become scarce is whatever it is that information consumes. And information consumes human attention.[14]

Remarkably, Simon made this observation in the 1970s, before social media sites like Twitter and Facebook, and before pop-up notifications. Those innovations have made his insight even more relevant. The challenge for the consumer is less about finding the money to purchase expensive content and more about finding the time and attention to consume it.

The problem of unlimited information competing for limited attention has been exacerbated by the Internet's dependence on advertising as its business model. So much of the content on the Internet is free to consumers, but it is ultimately paid for by advertisers. Big technology companies like Facebook and Google are, at their hearts, attention merchants, capturing attention and reselling it for profit.[15]

Nothing about this is new: it's what tabloid newspapers and TV channels have done for decades with advertisements and commercials.[16] And it isn't necessarily bad. But it is important to be honest about what is happening. When a company that sells shoes wants to expand, it aims to make and sell more shoes. When a company that sells attention wants to expand, it aims to capture and sell more attention. Ad-funded technology firms 'trade in users' eyeballs rather than subscriptions' and need their users to spend time on their platforms in order to make money.[17]

The result is that human attention has become one of the most sought-after commodities in the world. The cost of purchasing human attention increased by 7 to 9 times between 1990 and 2013.[18] And technology companies have become increasingly aggressive about competing for this scarce and expensive commodity. Often, the ultimate aim of these companies is to make using their website or app a frequent and automatic habit, and they've mined the insights of behavioural psychology to develop tactics to achieve such an aim. BJ Fogg, director of the Persuasive Technology Lab at Stanford University, has developed a model of behaviour change that has become widely used by developers who want to make their product habit-forming.[19]

Many of these tactics aren't intrinsically good or bad. Think about apps that track 'streaks', measuring the number of consecutive days you've performed a certain action. These are hugely motivating for anyone looking to start a new habit or give up an old one. They aren't a new idea, either: many schools employ a non-digital version of the streak by rewarding children who attend school every day in a term.

The language learning app Duolingo lets you build streaks that record how many days in a row you've logged in and practised your language, and many people like it because it incentivizes regular practice.[20] However, the social media website Snapchat uses the same tactic to get users to send a message to each other every day, which has gained criticism for being manipulative and even addictive.[21]

Another tactic is to remove all the friction associated with using a website so that it is as simple and easy to use as possible. Again, this has pre-digital antecedents: buying fruit and vegetables and placing them in a prominent position in your fridge or kitchen reduces the friction associated with eating healthily because it means healthy snacks are immediately available when you feel hungry. But removing digital friction can be used in ways that make people uneasy, such as YouTube's autoplay feature which automatically loads a new video when the previous one has finished, making it easier for people to get distracted from their original purpose.

Other tactics exploit our desire for novelty and social relationships. The 'like' buttons on many websites deliver what is called an 'intermittent variable reward'.[22] After you've posted a photo on Instagram or an update on Twitter, you can never be quite sure how many people will like it or repost it. This uncertainty keeps us checking and checking more than a more definite reward would, and the number of likes and clicks seems to be almost a measure of our popularity or social status.[23]

The sensationalist and extreme tends to grab attention more than the nuanced and deliberative. A former YouTube engineer showed how the site's algorithm gradually ratcheted up the extremism of recommended videos, so that a viewer who started out watching mainstream conservative or liberal videos would end up watching videos about political conspiracy theories if they let the autoplay facility run on.[24]

All of these methods have been supercharged by the vast quantities of data available to big technology firms that can easily trial different tactics, monitor their success, tweak, and repeat. Deep Mind, a division of Google, has developed AlphaGo, a sophisticated artificial intelligence programme. AlphaGo defeated one of the world's best human players at the board game Go, a landmark victory given the difficulty and complexity of Go. After this triumph, AlphaGo was redeployed by Google to improve the algorithm that selects autoplay YouTube videos.[25] One of the world's most powerful artificial intelligences is being used to persuade you to spend more time watching YouTube videos.

On most devices, even if you aren't actively browsing the Internet or using a connected application, you are at risk of being interrupted by a notification, with its noise, bright colours, and pop-up banners. This is especially the case with mobile phones, which are particularly designed to be distracting, such that accessing a website through a browser on a desktop is a different experience from accessing the equivalent application on a mobile.

> As more people began to access social media services on their smartphones, the attention engineers at these companies invested more resources into making their mobile apps stickier…some of these engineers' most ingenious attention traps—including the slot machine action of swiping down to refresh a feed, or alarm-red notification badges—are mobile-only "innovations".
>
> Newport, C., 2019, p.223

These are great examples of the differences between a mobile and a desktop computer.

Ultimately, when we use a connected device, we are using a device that is plugged into a distraction engine. Even if we are not actively using the device to browse the Internet, the notifications, beeps and pings are a frequent distraction and a reminder of what we might be missing out on.

How do students use devices?

What's the impact of these attention-grabbing design choices? Can students filter out these distractions or do they weaken their ability to learn? Or, is it possible that these distractions might be positive, allowing students to juggle competing sources of information and process them in a more sophisticated way than previous generations? Let's look at some research studies on how young adults use their devices, both for education and more generally. The participants in these studies range from primary pupils up to undergraduates. I will specify ages wherever possible, and use the term 'young adults' or 'students' as a catch-all.

Young adults spend a significant part of their day using devices. The UK media regulator, Ofcom (The Office of Communications), carry out frequent surveys into children's media use. In 2019 they found that 99%

of 12–15-year-olds spend an average of 20.5 hours per week online, 89% use YouTube, 83% have their own smartphone and 63% have their own social media profile.[26] On a wider geographic scale, in 2015, the OECD (Organisation for Economic Co-operation and Development) found that, in its member countries: 91% of 15-year-olds have access to a smartphone at home, and on average they spend about 19 hours per week online at home – although large differences in ownership of digital devices and time spent online are observed between different countries and economies.[27]

Young adults also tend to use their devices to multitask, which is one response to the constant demands on our attention from the modern Internet economy. Media multitasking can be defined as 'engaging in multiple media activities simultaneously'[28], whether that involves watching TV while texting a friend, or flicking between answering an email in one browser tab while online shopping in another.[29] It can also involve using media while doing a non-media task, such as texting while talking to a friend in person.[30]

In 2014, a group of researchers at the University of Amsterdam carried out a large literature review of multitasking among young people from the ages of 12 to the late 20s and found that it was especially prevalent in these age groups.[31] One study of American children aged 8–18 found that by multitasking, they squeezed ten hours a day of media consumption into just seven actual hours.[32] Another study from 2017 showed that in their general daily use of their laptops, undergraduates on average switch from one window to another in their browsers every 19 seconds.[33]

Of course, that's just how young adults use devices generally. What about how they use them for study? We lack good data on how these devices are used in the school classroom. The literature review referred to above, from the University of Amsterdam, showed that most in-class studies are carried out on undergraduates, and those with younger children tend to focus more on their use of technology to study in the home.[34]

Still, the research on in-class undergraduate use and home-study use offers some useful insights. It suggests that these general habits of multitasking and rapid switching carry over into study. One detailed study of 263 young adults (aged 12–23) showed that in a 15-minute home study period, they spent only 10 minutes studying and switched tasks every 6 minutes on average.[35] Another study asked a group of young adults (aged 13–18 years) to self-report their levels of multitasking while studying: 50% reported using social networks while doing homework, and 60% reported texting.[36]

The more extensive research on how undergraduates use devices in lectures and private study is also revealing: one study found that when privately studying for online classes, only 1.5% of undergraduate students reported *not* engaging in any multitasking: 63% reported using Facebook, and 69% reported sending text messages.[37] Other studies have asked students to place screen recording software on their laptops, and monitored their media use during lectures: 94% of them used email during the lecture, and 61% used instant messaging.[38] Another similar study found that in a 100-minute lecture, on average, students spend 37 minutes on non-course-related websites.[39]

Is this a problem?

So, students clearly do multitask when they are using technology, but what impact is this having? The educator Marc Prensky contends that far from criticizing multitasking, we should welcome it. In a 2001 article, he popularized the term 'digital native' to refer to students who have grown up using the Internet and taking it for granted.[40] Other research suggests that digital natives are those born after approximately 1980; 'digital immigrants', by contrast, were born before this date and as such were not immersed in the modern Internet environment at an early age.[41]

Digital Natives are used to receiving information really fast. They like to parallel process and multi-task... They function best when networked. They thrive on instant gratification and frequent rewards. Digital Immigrants don't believe their students can learn successfully while watching TV or listening to music, because they (the Immigrants) can't. Of course not – they didn't practice this skill constantly for all of their formative years...Today's learners are different... Today's teachers have to learn to communicate in the language and style of their students.

Prensky, M., 2001, pp.2–3

However, the research doesn't back this up. In a 2017 paper, Paul Kirschner and Pedro De Bruyckere found no evidence to support the existence of a generation of digital natives who think in fundamentally different ways from their predecessors.[42] A 2017 meta-review found a negative relationship between academic performance and social network use among young people.[43] Extensive evidence shows that nobody is that good at multitasking.[44] Even a simple task like walking can be compromised by listening to music or texting.[45] Attempting to combine more complex tasks causes even more problems, even for experts: doctors make more mistakes when they multitask as opposed to when they focus on one task at a time.[46] Practising multitasking doesn't make you any better at it: one study showed that participants who identified as heavy multitaskers did worse on a task that required multitasking![47] The term multitasking may be unhelpful, as the research suggests that we are not capable of true multitasking. Instead, what we end up doing is 'task-switching'; that is, switching our attention back and forth between the two tasks in a way that makes performance on both slower and more error prone.[48–49]

And research focussed specifically on education and young people backs this up. The 2014 literature review from the University of Amsterdam on adolescent multitasking looked at three domains: cognitive control, academic performance, and socio-emotional functioning. It found a small to moderate negative relationship between media multitasking and all three domains.[50] On its own, this doesn't prove that multitasking is to blame: it could just be that those students who choose to multitask are generally less committed to their studies.

However, newer research is filling that gap with experimental studies where students are randomly assigned to a 'device' or 'no-device' group.

Case studies: devices vs. no devices

- In a 2016 study by Carter, Greenberg and Walker, students were allowed to bring devices to some sections of their course, but not to others.[51] They did better on the sections with no devices.

- In a 2018 study by Glass and Kang, students were randomly split into two lecture groups.[52] One group were allowed to bring devices to their lectures and use them if they wanted. The others received exactly the same lecture at a different time, but they could not bring a device to the lecture. The students in the 'no-device' class did better on the final assessment. Fascinatingly, students in the 'device' class who chose not to use devices still did worse on the final assessment, which suggests that just seeing other students multitask is distracting. The same pattern has been found in another study.[53]

- Research on the specific impact of mobile phones shows that they appear to be even more distracting than laptops. When undergraduates at the University of Texas were asked to do a series of cognitive tests, they did better if they left their phones in another room and worse if their phones were on the desk in front of them.[54] This effect held even if the phones were turned off.

In research on adults, Oulasvirta et al. found significant differences between smartphone and laptop use.[55] The participants in this study used laptops and smartphones in different ways. They used their laptops in a few relatively lengthy spells. But they used their smartphones in frequent, short bursts. However, these short bursts were so frequent that they still ended up spending double the amount of time on their smartphone as on their laptop. The researchers concluded that these participants were checking their phones in a habitual, almost mindless way, which is, as we saw earlier, the goal of many designers.

We can conclude from this research that the design choices made by many big technology companies are having their intended effect. It is hard for young adults to concentrate on something for a long time when they are on their devices, and their devices provide a constant source of distraction even when they are turned off. Even if a school is not recommending that students watch videos on YouTube, if the student knows it's only a click away that can still be distracting. Even the websites and applications that aren't trying to distract you are part of an ecosystem that is. It's clear, too, that this kind of distraction is bad for learning, as it promotes multitasking (or 'task-switching') and reduces the working memory resources going towards the topic being studied.

What's the solution?

What can teachers, schools and students do if they want to maximize the ability to learn given the reality of the current Internet economy? Here, I will discuss the value of four different strategies.

- First, we could make learning more fun so that it can successfully compete against the distractions on the Internet.

- Second, we could train students to self-regulate better and to manage their attention in the face of distractions.

- Third, we could ban devices.

- Fourth, we could adapt connected devices so that they promote learning rather than hinder it.

Let's consider each possibility in turn.

Make learning more fun

We could make learning more fun and more of a regular habit by using some of the tactics we've discussed. We've seen some good examples of this already: many apps let you build a 'streak' of days studying, collect points or badges and upgrade your online avatar.

However, on its own this is not enough. First, connected devices encourage scattered, fragmented attention. The challenge for educators isn't just to grab attention but to sustain it.

Second, perhaps the most potent methods of getting our attention are ethically dubious. They play on our insecurities about our relationships with our peers, or feed us outrageous or false information. Tristan Harris, a prominent critic of the modern Internet economy, has called such tactics a 'race to the bottom of the brain stem'.[56] Education needs to stand above such a dubious competition, particularly when young children are involved.

Third, we need to be wary of assuming that well-designed, high-quality and fun lessons will prevent distraction. This is not the case. It is possible to get distracted even in such a lesson.

For an example of this, remember one of the undergraduate studies we looked at earlier by Glass and Kang. It sorted students into two groups: one that could bring their devices to a lecture, and one that could not. Both groups received the same lecture, and the students with the devices got distracted and did worse on the final assessment. The problem here can't be with the quality of the lecture, because the 'no-device' group were given exactly the same lecture, and they all learned more. If the lecture was ineffective, then presumably the 'no-device' group would have got distracted too, just by different means.

The presence of technology makes it more likely students will be distracted. Of course we should strive to make lessons as fun and engaging as possible. But devices can cause distraction regardless of the quality of the lesson.

Train students to self-regulate

What about training students to regulate their attention more effectively? We saw in Chapter 2 that gaining background knowledge about a subject makes it more likely that you can learn independently from a torrent of information on a search page, and navigate an online text with lots of hyperlinks.[57] So perhaps some kind of training could help students respond more effectively to distractions.

However, dealing with distractions is far trickier than learning how to study independently. It is possible to learn how to study independently: it's just that the most successful tactic involves gaining specific content knowledge rather than the more popular one of doing independent projects.

But when it comes to dealing with the types of personalized and persistent distractions of the modern Internet, it's not clear that anyone, even an adult, is particularly good at it. Trying to manage distractions by multitasking isn't particularly effective. And when we look at the way adults respond to digital distraction, we find that many of them are reverting to far more aggressive tactics than just self-regulation: either banning devices outright or altering them to remove their most distracting features. Let's consider each tactic in turn.

Ban devices

We've seen a couple of studies showing that banning connected devices in undergraduate lectures can improve academic performance.[58–59] Probably the strongest case for a general ban is on mobile phones, which encourage frequent interruptions and notifications, not the kinds of deeper thought often needed in the classroom. A 2015 survey of secondary schools in England found that students in schools who had implemented phone bans did better on their GCSE exams than students in schools with no phone ban. The positive effects were particularly pronounced for disadvantaged students.[60] Still, we can't expect to ban all devices, all of the time, because we need a way of getting the benefits of the many useful educational applications and websites.

Adapt connected devices

One way of getting the best of what technology offers without all of the negatives is to adapt devices to eliminate distractions. Over the last few years, a number of professionals whose work depends on focus and concentration have taken this path.[61] We can see this in the success of blocking software like Freedom, Cold Turkey and Focus, which let you block certain websites for certain periods of time, or set time-limits for their use. You can also edit the default setting on many devices to eliminate some of the more distracting features like notifications and badges.

Web blockers could be used more extensively in schools, but perhaps in the longer term the better solution is for educators and technologists to think more seriously about designing devices that promote learning. The best kind of learning device might be a tablet or laptop that has no notifications as a default and that has easy-to-set lock modes that block the Internet. Learning apps could also automatically block the Internet and notifications when you are using them.

These types of changes would not be easy, particularly for devices that rely on cloud software to work, but we have to think seriously about them if we want students to use devices to learn.

We should also consider the value of single-purpose devices. Instead of students responding to a multiple-choice question on a phone or a tablet, they could do so with a remote-control panel that has no other functions, and therefore no other distractions. And not every lesson needs to feature a device. It's possible to get a great deal of value from a device without using it in every lesson.

The modern Internet economy

Unfortunately, many in education technology are unwilling to confront the reality of the modern Internet economy and to consider the benefits of locking devices or blocking websites. For an emblematic example of this, we can look at the Massachusetts Computer Using Educators network, an organization that provides advice to teachers on how to use technology effectively. One teacher asked how to adapt a Chromebook to restrict his students' Internet use. Their response is instructive.

> I had a teacher come to me with a specific issue. He asked if I knew of any extension to lock down the Chromebooks in his classroom so that his students won't be able to wander off to various sites while doing classwork. The Ed Tech Coach in me immediately thought...*that is not a tech problem, it is a classroom management problem.* I'm pretty sure he could see THAT look on my face so he went on to explain that his students had some unique issues and haven't learned appropriate-use so using the available Chromebooks with them could be doing more harm than good. At that point, I had to dial my judgement down to '0' and think about ways that he could support appropriate use as they were learning to better self-regulate.
>
> Cahill, L., 2019

After supporting the teacher with a technical solution, the adviser goes on to say:

> Let me take a minute to say that this method is in no way a substitution for teaching students about appropriate use of devices and digital citizenship OR creating learning experiences that are so engaging and challenging that students want to do nothing but work-away!
>
> Ibid.

According to this point of view, if students get distracted on their Chromebooks, it's the teacher's fault for not creating engaging learning experiences or teaching the students about appropriate use of devices.

Or it's the students' fault for having some 'unique issues'. This advice encourages children to use devices that have been designed to distract our attention, blames them when they do get distracted, and it doesn't even consider the responsibilities of the billion-dollar technology companies who use all the money, data and intellect at their disposal to engineer distraction.

If we are to teach students about 'appropriate use of devices and digital citizenship', we could perhaps start by explaining to them how the modern Internet economy really works, and that removing yourself from the influence of devices is not an admission of weakness, but a sign of strength.

Summary

 Devices aren't neutral: they change the way we think

Connected devices are designed to distract us, and distraction is bad for learning.

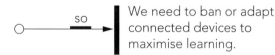

so

We need to ban or adapt connected devices to maximise learning.

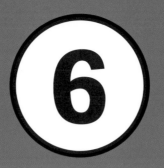

THE EXPERTISE OF TEACHING: CAN TECHNOLOGY HELP?

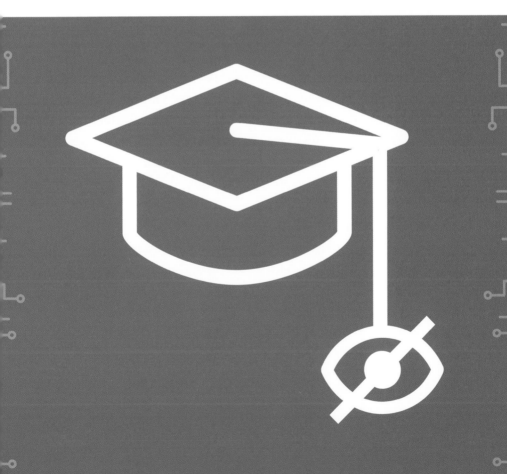

What about the teacher?

In my first year of teaching, I remember observing a lesson taught by my mentor on Shakespeare's *Romeo and Juliet*. She'd given me her lesson plan and a brief explanation of what she was planning to teach before the lesson. What impressed me the most about this lesson was that she seemed to have some kind of sixth sense about the questions the students asked and the difficulties they were about to encounter. Just as the class was getting ready to work in pairs reading a scene between Benvolio and Mercutio, she stopped and brought everyone back together. 'Remind me,' she said, 'what does Benvolio mean?' She'd told them this earlier in the lesson, so most of the class knew and could tell her that 'Benvolio' meant a 'well-wisher' or 'peacemaker'. 'Remember Benvolio is the peacemaker,' she said.

Initially, I was surprised by this intervention. Why had she stopped everyone at that point to ask that question? But as the class started reading out the scene in pairs, it quickly became clear. In this scene, Mercutio spends a long time unjustly accusing Benvolio of being hot-headed and quick to temper. But it's Mercutio himself who is hot-headed and angry, a character trait which has tragic consequences.

By reminding the students of Benvolio's actual character just before this scene, she was reminding them of the basic character dynamic of this scene. And as the students began reading the scene, it was easy to see how without that quick reminder, they'd have got confused and taken Mercutio's insults at face value.

I even saw one student break off in the middle of reading the scene to say, 'Remember, you're supposed to be the peacemaker!' My mentor's brief intervention only took a few seconds, and it wasn't even in the lesson plan. And yet it had clearly staved off potential confusion, and helped the students understand the scene and the play more deeply.

This anecdote reminds us of an important factor that is left out of many discussions about education technology: the teacher, and the expertise the teacher possesses.

Over the course of just one lesson a teacher might make dozens of similarly quick, real-time decisions designed to build their class's understanding. They may not make the right decisions all the time, but it would at least seem worthwhile to think about what they are trying to achieve and the nature of their expertise.

And yet, many of the approaches we've looked at ignore the teacher's decision-making and assume that a student can make equally good judgements. Most of the popular interpretations of personalization assume that students can choose their goals and methods. 'Just look it up' assumes that students can choose what they want to look up and interpret the results they find. Project-based learning assumes that students can learn the salient features from complex problems. Underpinning all these assumptions is the belief that placing a powerful general-purpose computer in a student's hands is sufficient for them to learn, and that they will have no problems in deciding on the most valuable content to look at, or in choosing what to focus on.

However, we've also encountered a lot of technological approaches which *have* engaged with the difficult question of replicating a teacher's expertise. Adaptive systems are trying to provide real-time hints and tips, a bit like my mentor's nudge about the meaning of the name Benvolio. Videos and online resources are deliberately designed to promote understanding, and quiz systems sequence questions in order to make memorization easier.

Given all the research showing the difference between novices and experts, and the value of expertise, it is these latter approaches that are more likely to be successful.

The big question, therefore, is not whether expertise is important or not. It's whether technology is capable of providing expertise and, if so, in what ways.

In order to answer such questions, in this chapter we will look more closely at the nature of human expertise and how technology might help it. I'll argue that neither human nor technological expertise on its own is enough: we need both. In the next chapter, we'll look at the expertise associated with another important part of education – assessment – and consider in what ways technology can help there.

The expertise of teaching

Expert teachers have developed rich knowledge structures about classroom practice, and these allow them to understand more about what is going on in a classroom, to anticipate misconceptions, to make quick, real-time adjustments to a lesson plan, and to consider how students are progressing towards longer-term goals. They can take their own understanding of a particular concept or skill and transform it into actions and instructions that allow students to understand it too.[1]

One study found that expert teachers could quickly generate lots of different examples and respond to students' questions in ways that advanced the objectives of the lesson. By contrast, novice teachers found it harder to adapt their explanations in the moment, and when they did so they often ended up introducing wrong information.[2] Another study of science teachers looked at how they would plan a practical lesson, and it found that the experts, unlike novices, anticipated the possible misconceptions the experiment might introduce and came up with strategies to address them.[3]

Expertise also matters for classroom management. We all know the popular stereotype of a teacher with 'eyes in the back of their head', able to spot misbehaviour even when their back is turned. The research suggests there is something in this: when expert teachers observe a lesson, they notice more details and recall events more accurately than novice teachers.[4] Teachers' expertise is rather like that of the chess players and readers we've encountered in previous chapters. They have large bodies of knowledge about typical classroom situations stored in their long-term memory which helps free up space in working memory to notice aspects of the new situation they are facing.

A lot of this research is based on quite small studies, but it draws on a wider literature about the strengths and limitations of human expertise. Two of the important figures in this area are Gary Klein and Daniel Kahneman. Klein's work has focussed on how experts like firefighters and nurses make rapid and accurate decisions in the heat of the moment. Kahneman's research, by contrast, looks at the failures of experts. In 2009, Klein and Kahneman collaborated on a paper that tried to reconcile these two schools of thought by working out the limits of human expertise and the areas in which it can and cannot develop.[5]

They concluded that some environments are better for developing expertise than others. Humans can develop expertise in 'high-validity domains', which are ones that are regular enough to provide you with cues about what might happen next. In this context, 'regular' doesn't mean easy, or simple to understand. Nurses and firefighters encounter highly complex, uncertain and dangerous environments, but they can pick up on reliable cues that indicate a building might be about to collapse or an infant has an infection.[6]

The other important factor identified by Klein and Kahneman is practice. To become an expert, you need time to learn the relevant cues and practise the skill. The amount of practice needed to become an expert varies depending on the specific area, and not all practice is created equal. Experience on its own can only take you so far; practice has to be more systematic than that.[7]

When these two conditions are met, real experts can develop. Both Kahneman and Klein agree that firefighters and paediatric nurses fit in this category, and other research suggests that teachers share some characteristics of this expertise.[8] Teachers learn to recognize when students are struggling to understand something, and over time they will also practise the best kinds of responses.

However, this is not the whole story. Human expertise is not perfect. It has flaws and limitations, and the research in this area is relevant for teaching too. Let's look at it now.

Where expertise fails

Expertise-induced blindness

For a few years now, the UK mathematics teacher Craig Barton has run a game on his blog called, 'Guess the Misconception'. Teachers read a mathematics multiple-choice question taken from the Diagnostic Questions website and have to decide which misconception was selected by the greatest number of students. The teachers don't do badly, but their intuitions are not always right.[9] This chimes with broader research that shows expert judgement of the expected difficulty of exam questions does not always predict how difficult students actually find those questions.[10]

This is the problem of expertise-induced blindness we encountered in Chapter 3: when an expert knows something so well and so fluently that they forget what it's like to be a novice encountering the same problem.[11] Even experienced teachers, with a lot of insight into the errors children make, can simply fail to anticipate a particular error.

Fractionation of expertise

A second flaw is what's termed the 'fractionation of expertise', which is when an expert can be good in one area but not in another closely related area. Doctors can be good at making some diagnoses, but not others. Weather forecasters are better at forecasting temperature than hail. And financial analysts might predict the commercial success of a business, but that's not the same as judging whether the shares of that business are under-priced.[12] This type of fractionation has been observed in teachers too, when they teach a topic or skill they are unfamiliar with.[13] My mentor could produce a well-timed question when teaching *Romeo and Juliet* not just because she understood her students, but because she understood the play. She might not have been able to make a similarly telling intervention on a play she'd never taught before.

The importance of feedback

Klein and Kahneman both emphasize the importance of quick and rapid feedback in developing expertise, but they also point out that in many professions, feedback is lacking because some of the behaviours we are trying to encourage are long-term, and we will not be around to gather feedback on whether what we did worked or not.[14–15] This is true of teaching: the ultimate aim of teaching is for our students to use what they have learned in school later in life, but we aren't around to gather data on that, so it's hard for us to establish a link between our teaching and what works in the long term.

There are further problems with feedback. So-called 'wicked problems' are those where the immediate feedback you get is misleading, as in the case of a doctor who made accurate predictions about which of his patients would develop typhoid.

> He confirmed his intuitions by palpating these patients' tongues, but because he did not wash his hands the intuitions were disastrously self-fulfilling.
>
> Kahneman, D. and Klein, G., 2009

A similarly wicked problem in education may be determining if a student has learned something or not. As we saw in Chapter 4, a student's performance on a task is a readily available and instant piece of feedback, but this performance is not the same as learning. Cramming for an exam is misleading because it produces high levels of performance in the short term, but not in the long term. This gap between immediate feedback and learning actually taking place may be one of the reasons why spaced repetition has never caught on, despite all the evidence in favour of it.

Expert bias

Experts can also be subject to bias. This is perhaps seen most significantly in interview situations, where irrelevant information about the gender or ethnic background of a job candidate can affect the decisions of the interviewer. For example, in the 1970s and 1980s, American symphony orchestras introduced blind auditions which led to more women being employed.[16] In education, this kind of bias is present with teacher assessment, and we will look at it in more detail in the next chapter.

More broadly, human judgement can be inconsistent.[17] Not every teacher makes excellent decisions every time. Not every doctor makes the right diagnosis every time. Factors like fatigue and hunger can affect our decisions.[18]

How can technology help?

The strengths and weaknesses of human experts that we have reviewed here are not unique to teachers, and if we look at other fields we can find ways in which technology has been used to address these weaknesses. In particular, algorithms are often used to provide the consistency which humans can lack.

Although we are accustomed to thinking of algorithms as something involving computers, at its most basic an algorithm is just a list of instructions. The anaesthesiologist Virginia Apgar developed an algorithm that could be used by midwives to determine whether a newborn baby was breathing properly.[19] One researcher showed that a simple algorithm – frequency of lovemaking minus frequency of quarrels – predicts marital stability better than the expert judgement of a marital counsellor.[20–21]

But of course, we are more familiar today with algorithms that are programmed into a computer and work automatically. Take finance: decisions about credit applications that used to be made by bank managers with a personal knowledge of the applicant are now made by computer algorithms that combine information about how many credit cards you have had in the past, whether you've ever missed a payment and how much of your available credit you tend to use.[22] These are examples of rule-based algorithms which consist of explicit and logical steps that have been written by a human.

These algorithms are not right all the time, but they will often do better than the human alternative. In particular, they'll be more consistent than a human. A loan applicant applying to two different branches of the same bank might get a different response. Indeed, a loan applicant applying to the same manager at the same branch might get a different response depending on the time of the day they see the manager and whether the manager has just accepted or denied a string of other applications. That won't happen with an algorithm: if it's given the same application, it will provide the same response.[23]

The roots of this approach lie in the work of Paul Meehl, a psychologist who wrote a paper in 1954 reviewing evidence from 20 other studies that showed statistical predictions were better than those of human experts.[24] Meehl's paper caused a great deal of controversy at the time, but it has been vindicated by subsequent research and by the way that algorithmic and statistical judgements have taken over so much of our world.[25] It is algorithms which decide whether we should be accepted for a mortgage or financial product, which prisoners should be paroled and which route we should take when we are driving somewhere for the first time.

To sum up, human teachers have strengths and weaknesses, and algorithms in particular may offer a way to address some of those weaknesses, particularly those involving inconsistency. In the rest of this chapter, we'll look at what the practical implications of this research are. I'll argue that we cannot rely solely on either technological or human expertise. Instead, we have to find a way of combining them.

Why we need humans

Given the power of technology, its consistency and its relatively low cost compared to human expertise, some would predict and indeed advocate for greater use of technology in schools. Back in 2008, Clayton Christensen predicted that 50% of US high school courses would be delivered online by 2019.[26] This clearly hasn't happened, but might it one day?

One barrier in the way of this prediction coming true is that so much education technology is not designed to promote learning. But suppose we could adapt tablets and laptops in a way that prevented distraction, and produce high-quality adaptive content and quizzes for every school subject. Even then, it's not clear that the majority of lessons could be delivered online, with little need for a teacher or a school, because human teachers provide important academic and non-academic benefits that are hard to deliver with technology alone.

Academic learning and in-person relationships are perhaps less separable than we might think. Young infants can pick up the sounds of a foreign language when they hear them from a real person. But when they hear exactly the same sounds on a video or tape, they don't learn as much.[27] Teachers provide motivation and supervision and, in many ways, they embody learning: imitating adults and sharing their attention are important mechanisms for learning.[28] Many people will have memories of how they came to enjoy and study a subject because the teacher of that subject showed an interest in them as a human being.

Even for adults, separating content and personal relationships is not straightforward: many relationships are based on shared interests. And personal relationships may be vital for communicating tacit knowledge, which consists of all the things we know how to do but find it hard to explain explicitly. The concept of tacit knowledge was first developed in the 1950s by Michael Polanyi. His classic example of a skill which we can possess but still be unable to explain is that of riding a bike.

> If I know how to ride a bicycle or how to swim, this does not mean that I can tell how I manage to keep my balance on a bicycle, or keep afloat when swimming. I may not have the slightest idea of how I do this, or even an entirely wrong or grossly imperfect idea of it, and yet go on cycling or swimming merrily.
>
> Polanyi, M., 1966

Tacit knowledge can also refer to the kinds of unspoken habits and practices that apprentices might learn from a mentor. The concept of tacit knowledge has become of great interest to computer scientists and philosophers in a range of fields because computer systems struggle to understand and replicate it, and so it suggests a possible limit to the capabilities of artificial intelligence.[29] We will look more at this in the next chapter, when we consider the difficulties involved with assessing essays.

Personal relationships matter for non-academic aims too. Students go to school not just to learn academic content, but to learn how to be adults, and the presence of peers and teachers is vital for this process. Of course, social media shows us that it is perfectly possible to socialize online, but a growing body of research shows us that online socializing is not the same as in-person.[30] In her book *Alone Together*, Sherry Turkle shows how many teens prefer to text than to talk in person because texting allows them to edit and prepare their response, unlike in-person conversations where they have less control.[31]

It is only fair to note that plenty of technologists are aware of the social nature of learning and are coming up with increasingly complex systems that attempt to copy human expertise in these areas. For example, the latest social robots interact with children in a more human and lifelike manner.[32] And in 2016 Apple acquired Emotient, a start-up which uses artificial intelligence to infer people's emotional states by analysing tiny changes in their facial expressions.[33]

Further developments in this area are almost inevitable. Online courses could be combined with social robots, emotion recognition systems and digital incentives. But we need to consider not just whether a new approach is possible, but if it is desirable. A computer may be capable of doing something, but we may still choose not to use it, or choose to continue developing human skill in this area. As we saw in Chapter 3, computers can record more accurate images than humans, but we still teach children to draw. Similarly, even if digital systems were capable of analysing emotions, we might still want humans in the classroom.

We also need to be careful not to define efficiency in a narrow way. For an example of this, consider the difference between writing by hand and using a word-processing programme. Word-processed documents are easier to read than handwritten ones, and it's more convenient to edit and share them. As a result, word-processing programmes have displaced handwriting in many workplaces. So when we look at paper textbooks and exercise books in schools, it's easy to dismiss them as old-fashioned clutter, and to think that for a more efficient classroom we should move everything on screen. But there is compelling evidence that writing by hand has important cognitive benefits for both children and adults; learning to handwrite helps children learn to read, and for adults, taking notes by hand builds stronger memories than typing notes.[34–35] If we moved everything in school on-screen, we'd miss out on these benefits.

Similarly, if we take a narrow view of efficiency then we might look at the genuine benefits of an online adaptive mathematics course and conclude that human teachers are unnecessary. But a broader view might conclude that while online courses can add a lot of value, they can't provide everything a human can.

Why we need technology

Given the patchy record of technology in education and the dubious interventions by big technology companies, some would argue that we should keep technology out of education as much as possible. But there are important reasons why we have to try and gain real benefits from technology. The main one is that there is increasing demand for good education, and our current methods of delivering it are already stretched.

In the developing world, there aren't enough schools and teachers. Even in the developed world, there are still some teacher shortages and big variations in quality. Data from the OECD's PISA survey shows that the biggest variations are not between schools, but within schools.[36] This in-school variation has different causes: one is that the background of individual students has a big impact on their performance.

However, another big cause is that teacher effectiveness varies. Teachers are not commodities, and they do not all have the same impact.[37] And even within one individual school, the quality of teaching will vary. Indeed, it is likely that even in those prestigious institutions that pride themselves on their bespoke brilliance, significant inconsistencies persist. And if it is hard for a leader to ensure consistent quality of teaching across one school, it is even more challenging to ensure quality across entire school systems. Simply employing more teachers doesn't have the desired effect either, as the following case study will show.

Why hiring more teachers and reducing class sizes isn't effective

The classic example of this is from the state of California, which in the 1990s invested billions of dollars in recruiting more teachers and reducing class sizes. However, attainment didn't improve as expected.[38] In order to reduce class sizes, California had to recruit thousands of new teachers. But not all of these teachers were as good as the established teachers, so the overall quality of education declined. While class size matters, the effectiveness of teachers matters too. Ultimately, this reform didn't have the desired effect because while it is relatively straightforward, if expensive, to increase the number of teachers in a system, it is harder to increase the number of *high-quality* teachers in a system.

Essentially, the challenge is to scale up quality teaching without reducing its quality. The word 'scale' is often treated as a dirty word in education, conjuring up images of 'factory' schools. There seems to be something about it that cuts against the humanistic ideals of education. Many of the world's most prestigious educational institutions make a virtue of their lack of scale, of their small size, and of the bespoke education they can provide.

But I hope we can see from the discussion above that far from being something to be feared, scale is something we desperately need. Let us just imagine what a world is like where we do not have reliable and effective methods of scaling up quality practice. The result is not that we have thousands of independent boutique schools all catering ideally for the niche needs of every individual child. Rather, it is that we have a limited supply of quality schools and quality teaching and no reliable way of increasing that supply to match the demand for it.

And the consequence of that is increasingly bitter political arguments about the best way to allocate such a scarce resource. Policymakers are then essentially reduced to deciding how this limited supply should be allocated: in a free-for-all, where wealthy parents buy up the best resources? We can probably all agree that we should have something fairer than that, but there are different definitions of fair. Should we allocate the best teaching to the poorest children or to the children who struggle the most with learning? Whomever we decide to prioritize, we are stuck in a situation where good education for one child means less good education for another.

The solution is to find ways of scaling up quality practice. This does not necessarily have to involve technology, of course. But the major advantage that technology has over humans is its consistency and replicability, and technology also has a track record of providing innovative leaps that allow for dramatic improvements.

Take printing, for example. Before the invention of the printing press, books were extremely expensive and scarce. A monk or nun could produce one double-sided page of manuscript in a day. The very earliest printing presses needed a team of four to produce 1,500 double-sided pages in a day, which is an almost 400-fold increase in productivity.[39] The invention of recorded sound allowed many more people to hear the works of great musical performers. And the invention of film allowed millions to see the work of great actors.

We can persist with the strategy of recruiting and training more people to do the job in the same way as before. But after a certain point, this gets harder and harder to do and not just because it is expensive, but because it runs up against natural limits: providing every child with their own on-demand qualified personal tutor in every individual school subject, for instance, would require more tutors than children! This kind of scaling is as if Gutenberg had decided to increase book production by employing more monks, or as though Edison had decided to increase access to music by building bigger concert halls. It would be literally impossible to produce all the books in the world today if they were handwritten.

Adaptive systems, quizzes and well-designed digital content have the advantage that they are replicable at scale. Indeed, the more people use them, the more powerful and useful they become as they gather data from more and more users, more than even the most experienced teacher can gather in a lifetime. What we have to try to do is to find a way of adding their benefits to the classroom without losing the benefits of human interaction. The next part of this chapter will consider some practical ways of doing this.

Combining technology and teachers

Perhaps the simplest way of using technology is to keep a relatively rigid distinction between technology and class teacher, and hand over to technology those tasks which students already complete outside the classroom. The obvious candidate is homework and independent study. Schools already set homework and expect students to study independently, so using technology for this doesn't reduce the role of human teachers at all. This approach also eases the institutional challenge of integrating an online curriculum with a classroom one.

Some programmes have been specifically designed to replace homework or independent study in certain subjects. They use adaptive questions so that different students get a different set of questions based on their individual strengths and weaknesses. One mathematics programme consists of hundreds of videos and thousands of practice questions which replace and mark the mathematics homework that a teacher would have set.[40] Teachers need to be trained in how the system works, and they deliver one lesson at the start of the year to their class demonstrating how the platform works. After that they can use the platform to set homework, check its completion and, if they wish, analyse the data on their students. This programme is aimed at schools, but other systems are aimed at parents.

Another online adaptive mathematics programme is designed to be used for 15 minutes a day by children aged between 4 and 14.[41] In 15 minutes, it is possible for students to answer and get feedback on dozens of questions that are pitched at the right level of understanding. Another independent study programme is designed for A-level students in certain subjects.[42] It provides videos and quizzes linked to specific exam boards, and personalized routes through this content.

One could also class certain online language learning platforms in this category.[43] They are not targeted at school students, but they certainly can be used by them as a supplement to in-school learning.

The advantage of these systems is simplicity. They all use complex technology, but they are all designed to be as straightforward as possible for the student to use, and it's clear to parents and teachers exactly how they should be used. In one way or another, they also all offer powerful adaptive technology that personalizes the content or questions a student receives. If a teacher, student or parent does want to use them in a more advanced way, then they can do so by analysing the performance data.

One reason these systems are easy to use is that they provide both content and an adaptive platform. However, for teachers who want to use the power of adaptivity but with their own content, there are other options. Plenty of digital flashcard programmes use spaced repetition algorithms to sequence practice in the best way, and many of them allow you to create your own flashcards as well as downloading pre-made sets.

Some adaptive platforms don't come loaded with any content. Instead, they allow teachers or groups of teachers to add or create their own content.[44] Then, as students progress through the content, the system records how well each individual is understanding each topic and adapts the content and questions they will see next accordingly. Organizations that have pre-existing large bodies of content can therefore use it to make them adaptive: for example, some of the quizzes on a popular UK revision website, BBC Bitesize, use an adaptive platform like this.[45] Schools, or groups of schools, can also use the platform to host their own content.

Programmes that use spaced repetition algorithms are an ideal way to use technology for two reasons. First, they directly address the flaw in human thinking that mistakes short-term performance for long-term learning. Second, they make personalized quizzing practical in a way that it isn't when humans have to constantly calculate and update the ideal spacing for many different questions and students.

Other promising ways of using technology focus less on the direct impact on students and more on ways of improving teachers' understanding. The thousands of student responses to questions on the Diagnostic Questions website[46] can help teachers learn more about their students' thinking. These questions are not adaptive, but teachers can use the insights from the national data and their own class's performance to improve their planning and teaching.

Systems that require teachers to create their own content, or change the way they teach, will require more work to set up and implement, but they have the potential to lead to greater changes too.

Future developments

It would be possible to combine many of these different approaches and create a digital learning system that would include curriculum-linked content, quizzes, an adaptive engine, and authoring tools for teachers to add their own content. Students could access this content through devices that have been adapted to minimize distractions from the Internet, and teachers could also access it for use in class.

If we pursued this vision, then on the surface, relatively little might change. The teacher would still be responsible for leading the learning of a group of students in a class. We could even choose to eliminate the use of connected smart devices completely in class. Video explanations could be delivered, when necessary, on the screen at the front of the class. In-class quizzes can be taken on paper and scanned in later, or they can be taken using clickers (dumb devices which record a student's choice and relay it to the teacher and learning system for analysis). There would still be time for in-class debates and discussions. The full benefit of adaptive quizzing could be deployed in homework tasks, or in a couple of selected lessons across the week.

However, behind the scenes, the adaptive quiz system would make automatic decisions about what a student should be quizzed on next. The insights from the system would be shared with teachers too, because the data from a quiz system can help teachers develop their understanding of how students learn. It would be harder for individual students to fall behind, or for teachers to develop their own misconceptions about how well a class have understood something. Teachers would not spend as much time preparing content or questions. But they would spend more time thinking about how each individual student in their class had understood that content.

As well as influencing what happens in the classroom, this kind of data could be integrated with teacher training and professional development. At the beginning of this chapter I described my experience of watching a colleague teach *Romeo and Juliet*. After observing this lesson and teaching it three or four times myself, I knew the kinds of misconceptions to anticipate. But technology could accelerate that process: a teacher training course could present trainees with the top misconceptions about

Romeo and Juliet from thousands of students, get them to watch three different videos of teachers explaining the misconception and then see which one had been most successful in resolving it.

However, the challenge with trying to integrate teachers and technology in this way is that, as well as needing sophisticated technological tools, it also requires significant institutional and behavioural changes, which are not easy to bring about. This approach would probably require collaboration between schools, technology companies, traditional publishers and teacher training colleges, which all have different cultures and traditions.

Perhaps the only organizations with the resources and capacity to try something like this would be the big technology firms. But as we've seen, they are pursuing different agendas that are not likely to promote learning at all. So it may well be that this more comprehensive vision of technology in education is not likely to be realized any time soon.

Still, we've also seen that there are a number of existing education technology applications which are effective and can have a big impact. The table on the following page categorizes ways of using educational technology for different users with differing levels of time and effort. There are lots of quick and simple approaches that teachers and students can get started with straight away, as well as more ambitious projects for schools or groups of schools that can invest more time.

This table deliberately deals only with software applications, not hardware. As we saw in Chapter 5, the research on investments in hardware alone is underwhelming. All of the software applications I've discussed here can be accessed on desktops, and none of them require students to have their own personal device. A school with 1 desktop computer for every 10 students can provide each student with about $2\frac{1}{2}$ hours of screen time per week. That's enough to implement the approaches outlined above, most of which recommend an approach of little and often.

Making education technology work in different contexts

	Low time and effort	Medium time and effort	High time and effort
Parent/ carer or student			Analyse the data from a learning app to learn more about the student's strengths and weaknesses.
Individual teacher	Use a flashcard app with pre-made flashcards.[47] Use a homework or independent study programme that doesn't require normal lessons to change much.[48] Use screen monitoring software or app blockers to reduce the potential for distraction.	Use a flashcard app to create your own flashcards.[49]	Create digital resources using Mayer's multimedia principles. Integrate digital quizzing into a sequence of lessons, evaluate the effectiveness, and re-plan the lessons based on the insights.
School/ group of schools		Design a professional development programme that helps teachers create diagnostic questions, integrate them into their teaching and analyse the data from them.[50]	Use an online adaptive platform that doesn't come with pre-loaded content to host content in one or more subject areas.[51] Work with teacher training institution to integrate insights into training.

Most schools in the developed world have many, many more devices than this already. Data from the British Educational Suppliers Association (BESA) from 2017 showed that there was on average 1 computer for every 3 students in UK schools.[52] OECD data from 2012 reports on the number of computers available to 15-year-old students in the UK and puts the figure even higher, at 1 school computer for every 1.4 15-year-olds.

In all the countries in the OECD survey, schools had one computer for every 4.7 15-year-olds.[53] The same survey showed that 96% of 15-year-olds reported that they had a computer at home.[54]

In the developed world, there is not an access problem. Indeed, given the problems of distraction and multitasking, the problem is more likely to be that students have too much unsupervised access to the Internet. Any school or group of schools looking to invest in education technology might be better placed to invest in software applications and staff training than in yet more hardware.

The applications I've referenced above and in the footnotes are not intended to be exhaustive or unique. They are chosen to illustrate general principles. There are thousands of different applications of varying degrees of quality, and new ones are appearing all the time. Based on the research we've looked at so far, on the next page is a set of questions to help evaluate any new education technology programme.

The last point about evidence is crucial. Ultimately, what we also need is more evidence and feedback about the effectiveness of different programmes. Some environments provide us with clear feedback which we can learn from: when a bridge collapses or an aeroplane crashes, the failure is immediately obvious.[55]

Educational success and failure, by contrast, are not as immediate or clear cut. The immediate feedback a teacher gets can sometimes be misleading. And there are many other medium- and long-term goals of education where the feedback is unclear or even non-existent. We will probably never find out if our students use the algebra they learned at age 14 in interesting ways when they are 25. And even our existing academic assessments can promote cramming and short-term revision strategies, meaning that they are not always a reliable guide to what works either.

One potential way of improving this situation is to develop better methods of assessment, and there are ways technology can help here. This is what we will look at in the final chapter.

How to evaluate education technology programmes

1. If it talks about personalization, how does it personalize?

   ✗ On the basis of learning styles?

   ✗ Do students get to choose what to study and when?

   ✓ Does it adapt to a student's needs based on their responses to questions?

2. What content does it teach? Who has designed the content/who will be responsible for designing the content? What research principles informed the design of the content?

3. How will it help build long-term memories?

4. Is it online-only or accessible offline? What devices can it be accessed on? How can the risks of distraction be mitigated?

5. Is it designed to be used for independent study or integrated into a school curriculum?

6. What training will teachers and students need to use it?

7. What happens if students are studying something and don't understand it?

8. How often should it be used?

9. How are the data/results presented?

10. What evidence is there that it works?

Summary

Teachers have real expertise – and they have blind spots

▌ EXPERTISE

In some ways, technology can mimic this expertise, e.g. through adaptive systems that give hints and nudges the way a teacher would.

In other ways, technology can't replicate this expertise, e.g. the social aspects of learning, teaching tacit knowledge, providing motivation and support .

▌ BLIND SPOTS

It's hard for teachers to know if a student has learned something for the long-term. Spaced repetition algorithms and long-term data collection can give teachers new insights.

All human experts find it hard to be consistent. Technology can help provide consistency and scale.

so → We need to combine the expertise of teachers and technology.

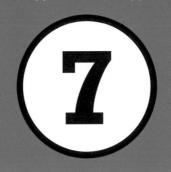

THE EXPERTISE OF ASSESSMENT: CAN TECHNOLOGY HELP?

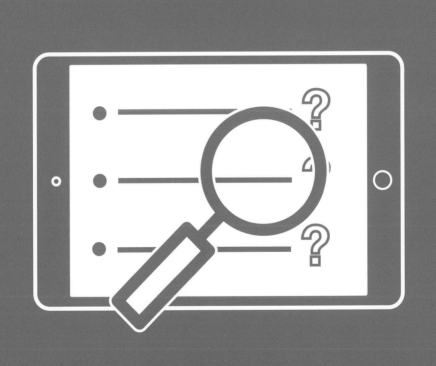

Can we trust assessment?

When I started teaching, coursework made up a major part of the GCSE English Language and Literature courses, a series of national exams taken by 15–16 year-olds in England. As a result, we had to be constantly on the lookout for plagiarism. Some was extremely easy to detect: I remember one boy submitting a four-page essay on *Romeo and Juliet* directly lifted from Spark Notes, a website that offers study guides for students. Quite apart from the totally different prose style, what really gave the game away were the adverts for teeth-whitening that he had copied and pasted from the website along with the essay.

But the potential plagiarism which worried me most was the reuse of essays from older students. This would be harder to spot than cut-and-paste jobs from the Internet, and it raised another concern: what if a student submitted an essay they'd copied from an older sibling, and I gave it a very different mark from the one it had originally received? I reassured myself that even if this meant they decided I was a lousy marker, they couldn't expose the discrepancy between the marks without revealing their own duplicity.

In fact, I probably shouldn't have worried. Or, at least, I should have worried about the whole system – not just me. Marking essays is tricky for everyone. One American study carried out exactly this experiment, by giving trained examiners the same essay to mark two years in row without their knowledge. The examiners had to grade the essays on a 6-point scale; only 20% of them gave the same mark both times.[1]

Larger-scale research also shows disagreement *between* markers. A recent study by the English exam regulator, Ofqual, showed that on a typical 40-mark exam essay question, there is a margin of error of +/–5 marks on average.[2] One major review of marking reliability showed that even experienced markers could struggle with consistency. In this chapter, we will look at the challenges posed by assessment and how technology can help improve it.

What makes assessment hard?

In the previous chapter, we looked at the problem of fractionated expertise, which is when someone can be an expert in one area but not in another closely allied area. This can explain some of the problems we see with assessment. We assume that someone who is good at teaching will be good at judging the quality of essays produced in their lessons. But that may not be the case. We saw in the previous chapter that expert classical musicians could still be biased against women when making hiring decisions. Teachers' assessments can also be biased, particularly if they know the students whose work they are marking.

Study after study shows that teachers tend to mark down candidates from ethnic minorities, from lower-income backgrounds, with special educational needs, and with behavioural problems.[3–7] When researchers compare the scores these candidates get in teacher assessments with the scores they get on exams, they find that teachers persistently undermark them.

Even when teachers don't know the identities of the students whose work they are marking, they can still be biased. For example, if you mark a set of 20 essays, changing the essay you begin with can often influence all of your later judgements; this is known as the anchoring effect.[8] The halo effect shows that on an exam paper with several questions, if a candidate writes a good answer to the first question, it can bias the marker's opinion of their later answers.[9] The neatness of a candidate's handwriting can affect the mark they get.[10] And we saw in the previous chapter that many different types of decisions can be compromised by fatigue or hunger.

In practice, I could see some of these problems in school. At moderation meetings, experienced teachers would disagree, often quite significantly, on the mark an essay deserved. Even colleagues who had taught for decades and marked for an exam board still found the process time-consuming and challenging. At times, the whole process could feel quite subjective, with extraneous factors like handwriting, the student's personality and essay length proving harder to dismiss than you might think. The same teachers who were capable of such rapid and accurate judgements in the classroom did not seem able to make similarly accurate judgements about students' work.

Sometimes, the accuracy of assessment is treated as a pedantic issue that's separate from the real business of education. But unless we have reliable methods of assessment, it's hard to know if our students are improving, if our lessons are having an impact, and if our teaching methods and curriculum choices are as good as they could be.

For me, as an English teacher, there were other reasons to be concerned about this issue. When I was at university, a typical insult offered by mathematics and science undergraduates was that English and the humanities were incredibly subjective areas where there were no right or wrong answers, and that as a result, a first-class degree in these subjects was not worth as much as one in mathematics or science. A lot of the time, my fellow literature undergrads would agree with this characterization and celebrate it: for them, the absence of a right answer was a sign of the superiority of the humanities.

I always found this argument dangerous. Perhaps it was true that in the humanities, unlike mathematics, there was more than one right answer. But no right or wrong answers at all? That felt like too extreme a proposition. And when I began teaching, I was even more convinced that this portrayal of English as a subject where anything goes was bad for its integrity. Why should any student bother trying hard in such a subject – and why should anyone care about such a subject at all?

Of course, this didn't mean that I wanted my students to produce cookie-cutter responses. I wanted to encourage them to have original and surprising opinions on literary texts. But as I showed in Chapter 5, these opinions depend on a solid understanding of the text. Without such a foundation, students wrote essays that were confused and contradictory.

Or did they? Here's where we hit the problem again: perhaps what I found confused and contradictory, others found original and surprising. If we can't agree on the worth of such essays, it's hard to agree on what type of education is best, or indeed if it is possible to say that any teaching method or curriculum is better than another. And while I felt certain that English and the humanities were more objective than people thought, I had to accept that the experience of having an essay marked, or marking one yourself, did not necessarily support this idea.

Improving assessment

Of course, there are ways of addressing these problems. Double or triple marking essays helps, but this doubles or triples the amount of time needed and so is hard to employ at scale either in schools or by exam boards.

Another response is to use more objective questions: markers do agree on the marks that should be awarded to multiple-choice questions or closed questions with just one right answer. These types of assessments can even be marked by machine, removing the possibility of human error. And while these types of questions are often stereotyped as being trivial and simplistic, they can be designed to assess quite sophisticated skills and often correlate quite well with scores on extended writing tasks.[11]

Closed questions have other advantages too. Using them allows test designers to construct adaptive tests which present different questions to different candidates depending on their previous responses.[12] These tests operate on a similar principle to the adaptive learning systems we saw in Chapter 2. If you get a question right, you get a harder question up next; get one wrong, and you get an easier one. The most sophisticated versions have banks of thousands of questions. They are quicker and more accurate than paper tests because students don't have to waste time answering lots of easy questions or skipping lots that are too hard.[13]

Still, closed questions can't solve all of our problems. Tests have an impact on how we teach, particularly high-stakes tests that have significant consequences attached to them. If writing was only ever assessed with closed questions, the risk is that it would end up only being taught with closed questions too. Lessons would be distorted and, over time, the correlation between performance on closed questions and on extended writing tasks could start to break down: students who did well on the closed questions might not be able to write good extended pieces.[14]

Not only that, but in many subjects, the essay is a vital part of the discipline. If we did use only closed questions in the assessment of English and the Humanities, we'd essentially be conceding the point about subjectivity, and agreeing that a major part of the output of English and the Humanities is not reliable enough for educational purposes. Ultimately, I did not think this was the case and I did think that teachers agreed more about writing than a typical moderation meeting might suggest. I was convinced that there was such a thing as good writing and analysis. We just had to find a better way of measuring it.

Can algorithms make the assessment of essays more reliable?

These problems seem like exactly the kind that can be solved by the consistency of algorithms, and there have been quite a few attempts to do so. Project Essay Grade (PEG) was an automated essay marker developed in the 1960s. Its creator, Ellis Page, began with a sample of essays that had previously been marked by humans. He then worked through the essays and identified about thirty different indicators that could account for their scores. Then, those features were turned into an algorithm that could assess new essays. The two most heavily weighted features were the length of the essay in words, and the standard deviation of the word length; other features were number of paragraphs, presence of a title, and number of apostrophes.[15]

PEG was very reliable. If you gave it the same essay on two different days, it awarded it the same mark, which is definitely not always the case with human markers. Not only that, but its marks did tend to correlate quite closely with those of human markers. If you took the average marks awarded by a group of human markers and compared them to PEG, PEG was closer to this average than any individual human marker.[16] So you could argue that PEG was more reliable than any individual human.

On the surface, this is another vindication of Kahneman and Meehl's predictions about algorithms outperforming humans. Even a fairly simple algorithm weighted towards the length of an essay can outperform human markers. However, it's not hard to spot what the problem is here, and to see why, half a century after its invention, this kind of marking hasn't eliminated the human kind.

Once teachers and students know that the algorithm rewards length, they will be encouraged to write more and more, even if this results in essays that are nonsense. In a 2001 paper, a group of researchers were challenged to see if they could fool a similar machine scoring system. The most successful cheat was an essay consisting of the same paragraph repeated 37 times.[17] The fundamental problem here, and one that affects all kinds of algorithmic approaches, is to do with causation. A number of algorithms operate by spotting correlations and using those to make inferences. That's fine in some contexts, but in others it causes problems.

For an example of this, let's look at finance again. The increasing amount of data that's available on our shopping habits allows companies to spot valuable correlations. In 2002, an executive at a big Canadian retailer looked at how their credit cards were being used. Customers who used their credit card at a pool hall were more likely to miss a card payment than customers who used their card at the dentist. Customers who bought carbon monoxide monitors or premium birdseed were also unlikely to miss a card payment. Those who purchased a 'Mega Thruster Exhaust System' for their car were more likely to miss a payment.[18]

Something similar has been seen in the UK. One big insurance company cross-referenced their insurance data with data from a supermarket loyalty scheme and found that home cooks are less likely to claim on their home insurance. One particular item correlated with low claim rates: fresh fennel.[19]

In all these cases, the inference is that the purchase of certain items can reveal something about your character which is of interest to an insurer or bank. People who purchase carbon monoxide monitors are responsible and safety-conscious and therefore unlikely to miss a credit card payment. The insurance company inferred that people who cook using fresh fennel are perhaps more responsible and house-proud and therefore more likely to look after their possessions.[20]

Buying fresh fennel clearly does not *cause* you to become less accident-prone – and indeed, becoming less accident-prone does not cause you to go out and buy fresh fennel. What's most likely is that there is a third factor, perhaps a personality trait like conscientiousness, that causes people to have fewer accidents and buy more fennel.

For the insurance company, the absence of causation may not matter too much. Knowing that fennel and low claim rates on home insurance are correlated is still useful, even if they don't know what causes it. They can still use the information in their algorithm.

However, when it comes to marking essays, we can't just rely on correlations like essay length, because it is so easy for people to game the system and create essays that are long but not good. Something similar is starting to be seen with credit scores. We don't know of any insurance scams involving bulk purchases of fennel, but plenty of real-life websites offer tips and tricks that will improve your credit score in ways that won't really make you more creditworthy. As a result of this, some economists worry that people have become so successful at gaming the system that credit scores no longer reflect the underlying risk.[21]

Credit-scoring companies can respond to gaming by keeping some aspects of their algorithm secret, but this then creates more problems. If companies don't make information about their algorithm public, it means that consumers who have been unfairly given a poor credit rating don't know why this is the case, or how they can improve it.[22] And again, this is not a solution for education. We want students to know what it takes to do well on an exam, not for it to be a secret.

Comparative judgement: combining algorithms and human judgement

Comparative judgement offers a potential solution to these problems. As the Director of Education at No More Marking, a company that provides an online comparative judgement engine for schools, my biases are relevant. My claim is that comparative judgement is an exemplar of the way we can combine human and algorithmic judgement, but you'll need to bear in mind that I am not a neutral observer.

Comparative judgement is a method of assessing open-ended tasks like essays that depends on both an algorithm and human judgement. The human judgements are in a different format, though. Teachers are used to marking essays one at a time, looking at the rubric or mark scheme for guidance. With comparative judgement, teachers look at two essays alongside each other and judge which one they think is better. There is no mark scheme.

This tweak improves the accuracy of the judgement, because humans are better at making comparative judgements than absolute judgements.[23] This is true when judging essays, but also when judging other phenomena, such as height, temperature, pitch and colour.

Suppose I ask a group of people to estimate individually the height of one person standing in front of them. Each individual might get close, and some of them might be spot on, but it is unlikely they will all agree on the right answer.

Suppose the same group are asked to look at two people standing in front of them and to decide which person is taller. It is now likelier that they will all get the answers right and that they will all be in agreement.

A similar illustration of the principle can be seen in a game which is used on the No More Marking website.[24]

Which question do you find easier to answer?

1. Mark how purple this is out of 8, with 8 being the darkest and 1 the lightest.

2. Which purple is darker?

If you look at 8 different shades of a colour individually it will be very difficult to number them from 1 to 8 in darkness. But if you compare all the different pairs of the colour repeatedly you will end up with them in order from lightest to darkest, giving you a scale 1–8:

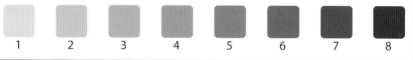

Comparative judgement eliminates many opportunities for bias to creep in. With absolute judgement, the anchoring effect means that the quality of the first essay you see has a big impact on how harsh or generous you are as a marker. With comparative judgement, because you only have to compare two scripts, this is not a problem. It's impossible to be a harsh or generous marker with comparative judgement: if you see two essays and think they are both terrible, you still have to select one as being better. And if you see two and think they are both terrific, you still have to choose one as being worse.

On their own, these judgements would not provide us with the assessment scores we need. What is needed is a way of combining all of the judgements, which is where the algorithm comes in. The comparative judgement algorithm was developed in the 1920s by an American psychometrician, Louis Thurstone, and it works by combining all of the individual judgements together to create an absolute scale.[25] In Thurstone's time, this process involved a lot of manual calculations, but modern software allows teachers to scan the scripts into their computer, do all the judgements online, and receive the results instantly.

To get reliable scores, you need to make a lot of judgements. In 2018, the English exam regulator, Ofqual, carried out a research project into AS-level History which found that carrying out four judgements per script provided reliability equivalent to traditional single marking.[26] Five judgements per script provided reliability equivalent to traditional double marking. The reliability kept improving as more judgements were added. No More Marking has run several large-scale national assessment projects which confirm these findings. Typically, it is recommended that a teacher needs to make ten comparative judgements per script: this provides reliability equivalent to a margin of error of +/– 2 marks on a 40-mark essay.

Ten judgements per script means that if you want to assess 100 students, you will need to make 1,000 judgements. This may sound like a lot, but each judgement can be made fairly quickly. In big judging projects, teachers take an average of 20 seconds per judgement. One criticism of comparative judgement is that it is not possible to make decisions this quickly, so teachers must be relying on features like handwriting that do not properly reflect the quality of the work.

However, we've seen from the literature on decision-making that in certain contexts experts can make rapid judgements that are still accurate. Speed does not necessarily entail a loss of accuracy. Comparative judgement simplifies the judgement process, removes the potential for lots of biases, and makes it easier for teachers to access and apply the knowledge they do possess about what makes good writing. It creates a context in which rapid judgements are more likely to be accurate.

Another criticism is that this process lacks transparency because it removes the guidance provided by the rubric. Perhaps the teachers are all agreeing, but without a rubric, we don't know what they are agreeing about. They may just be basing their decisions on handwriting or other superficial features of the writing.

This is an important question which goes to the heart of the challenges of marking essays. We do find generally good correlations between comparative judgement and marking with rubrics. Still, on its own, this is not enough: as we saw with the automated-scoring systems, high correlations do not prove validity. The automated scoring system agreed fairly closely with teacher judgements, but it did so by focussing on relatively superficial features of writing, not on true indications of quality.

As with the automated scoring systems, an interesting way of considering the validity of the comparative judgements is to look not at where the traditional assessments and comparative judgement agree, but at where they disagree. What types of essays do well with traditional assessments but badly with comparative judgement? And what type do well with comparative judgement but badly with traditional assessments?

Below are two such outliers, which are extracts from larger portfolios of writing:

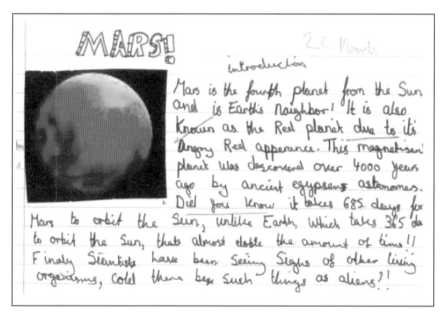

Script A performed well with comparative judgement, but not with the traditional assessment.[27]

Script B did poorly on the comparative judgement assessment, but better with the traditional assessment.[28]

In discussions with teachers, when asked which script they would like to see get the higher score, they almost unanimously agree with the results of the comparative judgement assessment. They feel that script B is coached and mechanical, whereas script A is more fluent and readable. Script B includes the range of punctuation specified by the rubric scheme, but that doesn't necessarily make it a better piece of writing.

Script A falls foul of the rubric's requirement for accurate spelling. However, this just shows the difficulty of attempting to assess spelling in open-ended tasks. Script A does feature misspellings, but some of them are quite difficult. There is no guarantee that the pupil who wrote Script B could spell them all. The fairest way of assessing spelling is to give all students the same spelling test. Assessing it through extended writing like this may end up not encouraging better spelling but discouraging ambitious word choice.

These two scripts illustrate just some of the challenges of marking with rubrics. Rubrics can be fairly general, or more specific and precise, but each type has its own problems. Holistic rubrics provide quite general statements about the type of work they expect to see: to get one grade your writing has to be 'fluent', and to get the next grade up it must be 'confident'.[29]

Such statements are so general that they are capable of being interpreted in different ways by different markers. A typical response is to tighten up the rubric, and make it more specific and precise. This is exactly what happened in England in 2015 with the national primary writing assessment: the rubric was made more specific to prevent some of the inconsistent interpretations of vague statements.[30]

However, not only does this not help markers to agree, but it introduces a whole new set of problems which are quite similar to the problems of automated scoring algorithms. England's new rubric required pupils to 'spell most words correctly', which on the surface, seems like the kind of useful and transparent guidance we want to give to pupils. In practice, as we can see from scripts A and B, it could equally well just have led to students being discouraged from using more ambitious vocabulary.

Other requirements can have equally unwanted consequences. My favourite example of this involves the statement on the rubric that requires the use of hyphens to get the top grade. One teacher told me that in order to make sure her pupils ticked this box, she had told them that the main character in all their stories should be 'Mary-Jane', who was aged 'twenty-two'.

These unintended consequences have been particularly visible in the English primary writing assessment since 2015, but they have been noted before in the literature.[31–32] 'Hyperspecific' rubrics define quality so narrowly as to preclude different legitimate approaches to the task, and distort instruction so that it only focusses on what is in the rubric. Ultimately, they defeat the point of having an open writing task in the first place by making the assessment 'more reductive, and thus limiting the room for creativity and critical thinking.'[33]

Ultimately, the reason why rubrics fail is because there is a limitation to what we can express in words. We saw in the previous chapter the concept of 'tacit knowledge': the ability to ride a bike or float in water, which we know how to do but can find hard to explain. Michael Polanyi notes that words and rules are not the best ways of communicating this kind of knowledge.

> Maxims are rules, the correct application of which is part of the art which they govern. The true maxims of golfing or of poetry increase our insight into golfing or poetry and may even give valuable guidance to golfers and poets; but these maxims would instantly condemn themselves to absurdity if they tried to replace the golfer's skill or the poet's art. Maxims cannot be understood, still less applied by anyone not already possessing a good practical knowledge of the art. They derive their interest from our appreciation of the art and cannot themselves either replace or establish that appreciation.
>
> Polanyi, M., 2012, p.32

Similarly, in attempting to reduce down the skill of writing to some maxims on a rubric, we end up with absurdities like 'Mary-Jane, the twenty-two-year-old'. If we wanted to make the skill of writing a good essay transparent, we would look beyond the rubric and instead at the curriculum a student experiences over their time in school. As discussed in Chapter 4, the skill of writing a good essay is best developed by learning from carefully constructed examples of good writing. Similarly, statements on a mark scheme cannot communicate the essence of good writing as well as carefully constructed examples of sentences and vocabulary can.

Still, while rubrics clearly have flaws, these do not prove that the results from comparative judgement are superior. More research is needed in this area, some of which we are carrying out. In an ongoing piece of research, we have recorded pairs of teachers discussing the reasons behind their judgements and the features they are basing the judgements on. Another possible area of research is to get professional writers who are not teachers to judge and see if their judgements agree with those of the teachers. This would help us to see if there is broader agreement about what constitutes quality writing.

The search for better methods of assessment is definitely worth it. Throughout history, methods that have improved measurement have ended up spurring innovation. The invention of the thermometer, watch and kilometre all had transformative impacts in related fields.[34] Algorithms on their own may not be able to assess quality, but when combined with human judgement they offer the potential of genuine improvements.

What about machine learning?

The similarities between the problems with rubrics and the problems with rule-based algorithms suggests that machine learning might help too. Machine learning is particularly useful in areas where it is difficult to write specific and explicit rules for an algorithm to follow, like driving cars, translating languages or deciphering handwriting. These are all areas where human expertise exists, but where reducing such expertise to step-by-step lists or rule-based algorithms has proved fiendishly difficult.[35]

Machine learning takes a different approach. A machine-learning algorithm will trawl through a large data set finding patterns and rules within it and use those to create a new algorithm that can then be applied to new data. To go back to our credit rating example, a company seeking to improve its identification of credit risks would provide its learning system with past data on customers who had and hadn't defaulted. The learning system would then use all of that data to spot patterns in what led to a customer defaulting and create an algorithm that could then be used to predict the default risk of a new customer.[36]

Such a system would seem ideal for assessing essays, as it avoids the problems with rule-based algorithms and rubrics that we have just encountered. Still, there are a couple of issues that should make us wary. First, the problems with correlation and causation that we encountered with rule-based algorithms are even more of a problem with machine-learning algorithms. This is because machine learners seek patterns in large data sets with lots of variables, so they can find patterns that don't hold true in the real world.

David Leinweber, a data scientist, illustrated this well by searching through a database of statistics to find one that could 'predict' the US stock market. He wanted to show that analysing huge amounts of data for patterns can lead to finding purely coincidental correlations between data sets. He found that combining data for butter production in Bangladesh, American cheese production and the population of sheep in Bangladesh 'explained' 99% of the stock-market variation between 1983 and 1999.[37]

The Spurious Correlations website has a whole collection of such oddities, showing strong correlations between the number of people who drowned by falling into a swimming pool and the number of films Nicolas Cage has appeared in.[38] These are extreme examples, but this problem of mistaking the noise for the signal, or 'over-fitting', is perhaps the biggest challenge to modern machine learning.[39–40]

Second, the workings of machine-learning algorithms can be difficult to understand, even for the designer.[41] With comparative judgement, it is possible to trace every result back to the decisions of individual humans. Machine-learning algorithms are often described as 'black boxes', because it's hard to know how they arrive at their decisions. This means that when there are errors and anomalies – and even a good system will not be perfect – it is hard to investigate them. Again, the impact this would have on a wider system is problematic. If students and teachers do not know what is being rewarded, or why it is being rewarded, it can have a negative impact on teaching and learning.

This does lead to some broader philosophical questions. One computer scientist has argued that far from machine learning systems being unaccountable, it is we humans who are unaccountable.[42] It *is* ultimately possible to unpick a machine learning algorithm and work out exactly why it made the decision it made. In many ways, humans are far more inscrutable. Of course, you can ask someone why they made a certain decision, and they can respond in good faith, but a lot of the time we don't know why we make certain decisions. The root causes can be hidden away beneath the level of our consciousness, and our public reasoning is more of a post-hoc justification than an actual explanation.

There may be some truth to this. But I still think that we are better off having human judgement involved in marking essays because, ultimately, we want our students to learn to write in ways that other humans appreciate. As long as we can ensure that human judgement is reliable, then it should be the final criterion, however inexplicable it may appear. And when we can find a way of making human judgement more consistent, it opens up possibilities of making it less mysterious. Ultimately, we have to use technology to uncover the mysteries of the human mind, not create new ones.

Summary

Assessing open tasks like essays is necessary but hard to do reliably

On their own, algorithms aren't good at asssessing open tasks: it's too easy to game their rules.

so

We need to combine the consistency of algorithms with the depth of human judgement. This is what comparative judgement does.

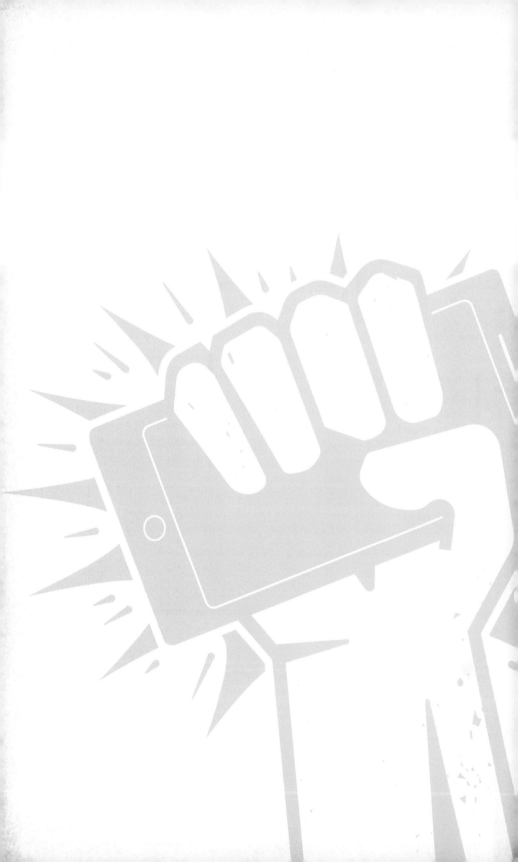

CONCLUSION: DISRUPTING EDUCATION

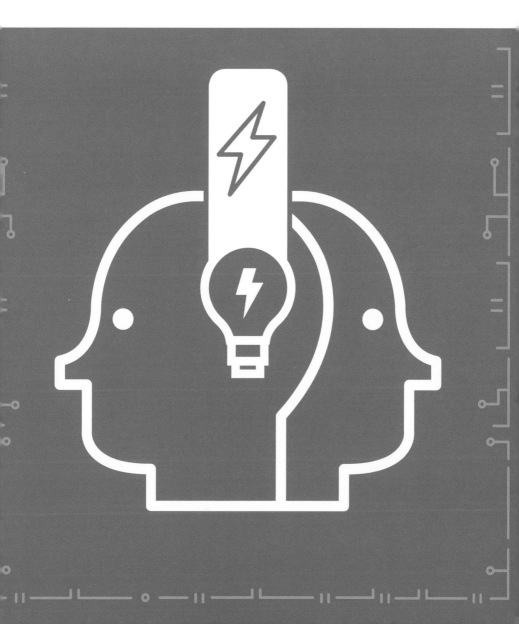

Disruptive innovation happens when a new technology provides a different way of fulfilling people's needs. The Internet means you can get your news via a computer screen, not printed on paper. Digital cameras make it easier for you to capture images without bothering about rolls of film. Cars let you travel between two places without a horse.

Because these innovations are so unexpected and powerful, existing customers and companies are often blindsided by them. As a result, disruptive innovators are often mocked as fantasists when they start out. If they do succeed, it's easy to assume that their success is due to unique imagination and vision rather than anything as mundane as customer research. Henry Ford is often quoted as saying, 'if I had asked people what they wanted, they would have said faster horses.'[1] Similarly, no profile of Apple's Steve Jobs is complete without reference to his 'reality-distortion' field which enabled him to persuade customers and employees to believe in his vision for technology.[2]

Undoubtedly, there is a lot of truth to this. Great innovators do have powerful imaginations and the ability to convince others of the truth of their vision. Still, the above examples show that great innovators are constrained by reality in important ways too. New inventions have to obey the laws of physics: iPhones and Fords are not powered by cold fusion. And they have to fulfil purposes that people want, even if people may not realize what they want. Ford did not ignore his customer's desire for a faster means of transport, he just interpreted it in a different way.

If we apply this insight to education, then we can see that any transformative educational vision still needs to be founded in two important realities. First, the reality of how human beings think and learn. Second, the reality of what schools, teachers, students, parents and wider society want from education.

The most successful innovations in education technology today are working within those constraints. They are finding ways for technology to help students learn challenging content in fun and efficient ways and revealing more about human cognition in the process.

But there are other cases where the concept of disruptive innovation has justified approaches which are built on little else but imagination. Personalization is too often interpreted as being about learning styles or student choice. The existence of powerful search engines is assumed to render long-term memory irrelevant. Active learning is about faddish and trivial projects. Connected devices are seen as a panacea for all of education's ills, when they may just make it easier for students to get distracted. Successful disruptive innovation solves a problem better than the existing solution. Too many education technology innovations just create new problems.

The dividing line between the more and less effective approaches we've looked at is in the attitude to teacher expertise. The more effective approaches seek out what is valuable about teacher expertise and try to copy or even improve on it. The less-effective approaches assume it is irrelevant or can be ignored. Ultimately, they promote a form of discovery learning that has been repeatedly tried and found wanting in the past. For all that 'looking it up on Google' has a superficial novelty to it, it is actually just a manifestation of discovery learning, an idea which has a long history of failure.[3]

Unfortunately, the big technology firms who govern so much of our online life are not on the side of the evidence. Still, we can't blame them for all our woes. First, it is not the technology companies who invented these bad ideas: many of them originate within education. Second, educationalists have proved unwilling to criticize or scrutinize the educational efforts of big technology firms. So it would be disingenuous to blame big technology companies for all of these problems: if they are promoting bad ideas, it's at least partly because we've made it easy for them to do so.

In the research I did for this book, I read many different explanations of why education technology has failed and what it would take to change that. If only there was more money, or better training, or more open-minded teachers, or schools that weren't designed to be like factories, then technology really could improve education.

However, ultimately I have concluded that more important than any of these factors is the power of bad ideas. If we assume that learning styles exist, that cognitive overload doesn't exist, that students can pick up knowledge as they go, and that attention is an infinite resource, we will never improve education, however much, or little, technology we use. If we persist with faulty ideas about how humans think and learn, we will just extend a century-long cycle of hype and disillusionment.

But if we can disrupt the influence of bad ideas, there are enormous opportunities for technology. Adaptive learning systems can provide more personalized teaching, spaced-repetition algorithms can make it easier for us to build long-term memories, and sophisticated uses of data can make assessment more precise and meaningful.

These evidence-based innovations offer the promise of a genuine educational revolution that could transform the way we learn and teach.

Endnotes

Foreword

1. Atkins, A., 2017. What is the Origin of "Clothes Make the Man"? 22 October. *Medium* [online]. Available at <https://medium.com/@alex_65670/what-is-the-origin-of-clothes-make-the-man-7f75e070bf45> (accessed 10 December 2019)

2. Krause, S. (2000). "Among the greatest benefactors of mankind": What the success of chalkboards tells us about the future of computers in the classroom. *The Journal of the Midwest Modern Language Association, 33*(2), pp.6–16. Available at <Doi:10.2307/1315198>

Introduction

1. OECD, 2015. *Students, Computers and Learning. Making the Connection.* Paris: PISA, OECD Publishing. Available at <https://doi.org/10.1787/9789264239555-en> (accessed 13 November 2019)

2. Cristia, J., Ibarraran, P., Cueto,S., Santiago, A. and Severin, E., 2012. *Technology and Child Development: Evidence from the One Laptop Per Child Program* (IDB Working Paper No. IDB-WP-304). Washington, DC: Inter-American Development Bank

3. Malamud, O. and Pop-Eleches, C., 2011. Home Computer Use and the Development of Human Capital. *The Quarterly Journal of Economics, 126*(2), pp.987–1027

4. Kitchen, S., Finch, S. and Sinclair, R. (Nat-Cen), 2007. *Harnessing Technology Schools Survey 2007.* Coventry: BECTA

5. Ofsted, 2004. *ICT in schools: the impact of government initiatives five years on.* London: Ofsted Publications Centre, p.3

6. Parkinson, Justin, 2004. £25m extra for schools technology. *BBC* [online]. 7 January. Available at <http://news.bbc.co.uk/1/hi/education/3375465.stm> (accessed 4 November 2019)

7. Cross, Michael, 2005. Chalk one up to the whiteboard. *The Guardian.* 6 October. Available at <https://www.theguardian.com/technology/2005/oct/06/elearning.education> (accessed 4 November 2019)

8. Kitchen, S., Finch, S. and Sinclair, R., 2007. *Harnessing Technology Schools Survey 2007.* Coventry: BECTA, p.36

9. Gillen, J., Keline Staarman, J., Littleton, K., Mercer, N. and Twiner, A., 2007. A "learning revolution"? Investigating pedagogic practice around interactive whiteboards in British Primary classrooms. *Learning, Media and Technology, 32*(3), pp.243–56

10. Hinds, D., 2018. Schools must Harness cutting edge technology to engage and inspire the next generation. *The Telegraph* [online]. Available at <https://www.telegraph.co.uk/education/2018/08/07/schools-must-harness-cutting-edge-technology-engage-inspire/> (accessed 13 May 2019)

11. Apple, 2013. *Apple Awarded $30 Million iPad Deal From LA Unified School District* [online]. June 2013. Available at <https://www.apple.com/newsroom/2013/06/19Apple-Awarded-30-Million-iPad-Deal-From-LA-Unified-School-District/> (accessed 12 May 2019)

12. Blume, H., 2017. U. S. Attorney Won't File Charges after Probe of $1.3-Billion iPads-for-All Project in L.A. Schools. *Los Angeles Times* [online]. Available at <https://www.latimes.com/local/lanow/la-a-me-edu-no-charges-ipad-probe-20170221-story.html> (accessed 12 May 2019)

13. Clarke, A. C., 1962. *Profiles of the Future*. New York: Harper and Row, pp.3–4

14. For example, see Camilla Turner, C., 2019. Replacing blackboards with interactive whiteboards was a waste of money, Education Secretary says. *The Telegraph* [online]. Available at <https://www.telegraph.co.uk/education/2018/08/07/replacing-blackboards-interactive-whiteboards-waste-money-education> (accessed 13 May 2019)

15. American Federation of Teachers, 2018. *AFT Resolution, Future of Teaching and Technology*. Available at <https://www.aft.org/resolution/future-teaching-and-technology> (accessed 13 May 2019)

16. For example, see Mahmood, A., 2018. How can the DfE use Edtech to reduce teacher workload?. *Schools Week* [online]. Available at <https://schoolsweek.co.uk/how-can-the-dfe-use-edtech-to-reduce-teacher-workload/> (accessed 13 May 2019)

17. Emerich, P., 2019. Why I Left Silicon Valley, EdTech, and "Personalized" Learning [online]. *Paul Emerich France*. 15 January. Available at <https://paulemerich.com/2018/01/15/why-i-left-silicon-valley-edtech-and-personalized-learning/> (accessed 13 May 2019)

18. Bowles, N., 2019. Silicon Valley Came to Kansas Schools. That Started a Rebellion. *The New York Times* [online]. 21 April. Available at <https://www.nytimes.com/2019/04/21/technology/silicon-valley-kansas-schools.html> (accessed 14 May 2019)

19. Walker, A., 2019. Technology leaders worry schools are not preparing their children for the future. *The Times* [online]. 8 January. Available at <https://www.thetimes.co.uk/article/tech-savvy-parents-worry-schools-are-not-preparing-their-children-for-the-future-r88phqpp3> (accessed 14 May 2019)

20. Lomazzi, M., Borisch, B. and Laaser, U., 2014. The Millennium Development Goals: experiences, achievements and what's next. *Global health Action*, 7(1), 23695

21. UNESCO, 2017. *Reading the past, writing the future: Fifty years of promoting literacy*. Paris: UNESCO. pp.21–3; p.26

22. Gurria, A., 2018. *PISA 2015 results in focus*. Paris: OECD Publishing, p.5. Available at <https://www.oecd.org/pisa/pisa-2015-results-in-focus.pdf> (accessed 14 November 2019)

23. Mullis, I. V. S., Martin, M. O., Foy, P. and Hooper, M., 2017. *PIRLS 2016 International Results in Reading*. Available at <http://timssandpirls.bc.edu/pirls2016/international-results/> (accessed 4 November 2019)

24. Mullis, I. V. S., Martin, M. O., Foy, P. and Hooper, M., 2016. *TIMSS 2015 International Results in Mathematics*. Available at <http://timssandpirls.bc.edu/timss2015/international-results/> (accessed 4 November 2019)

25. OECD, 2013. *Skilled for Life? Key findings from the survey of adult skills*. Paris: OECD, p.12

26. Hanushek, E. A. and Woessmann, L., 2007. *The Role of Education Quality for Economic Growth*. Working paper, No 4122. Washington: The World Bank

27. Flynn, J. R., 2007. *What Is Intelligence?: Beyond the Flynn Effect*. Cambridge: Cambridge University Press

28. Dutton, E., van der Linden, D. and Lynn, R., 2016. The negative Flynn Effect: A Systematic Literature Review. *Intelligence*, 59, pp.163–69, Available at <https://doi.org/10.1016/j.intell.2016.10.002>

29. OECD, 2017. *PISA 2015 results (Volume II) Policies and Practices for Successful Schools*. Paris: OECD, pp.185–86. Available at <http://dx.doi.org/10.1787/9789264267510-en> (accessed 4 November 2019)

30. Ibid., pp.204–7

31. Hirsch Jr, E. D., 2002. Classroom research and cargo cults. *Policy Review* [online]. October 1. Available at <https://www.hoover.org/research/classroom-research-and-cargo-cults> (accessed 4 November 2019)

32. McCorduck P., 2004. *Machines Who Think: A Personal Inquiry into the History and Prospects of Artificial Intelligence*, 2nd ed. Natick, MA: AK Peters (CRC Press)

1: The science of learning

1. Cedar R. and Willingham D., 2010. The Myth of Learning Styles. *Change: The Magazine of Higher Learning*, 42(5), pp.32–5, Available at <https://doi.org/10.1080/00091383.2010.503139> (accessed 14 November)

2. Miller, G. A., 2003. The cognitive revolution: a historical perspective. *Trends in Cognitive Sciences*, 7(3), pp.141–4

3. McCorduck P., 2004. *Machines Who Think: A Personal Inquiry into the History and Prospects of Artificial Intelligence*, 2nd ed. Natick, MA: AK Peters (CRC Press)

4. Moor, J., 2006. The Dartmouth College Artificial Intelligence Conference: The Next Fifty Years. *AI Magazine*, 27(4), pp.87–91

5. Newell, A. and Simon, H., 1956. The Logic Theory Machine – A Complex Information Processing System. *IRE Transactions on Information Theory*, 2(3), pp.61–79

6. Simon, H. A., 1996. *Models of my life*. Cambridge, MA: MIT Press, p.213

7. Sejnowski, T. J., 2018. *The Deep Learning Revolution*. [ebook] Cambridge, MA: MIT Press, loc. 1064–1257. Available at <http://www.amazon.co.uk/kindlestore> (accessed 4 November 2019)

8. Cowan, N., 2014. Working Memory Underpins Cognitive Development, Learning, and Education. *Educational Psychology Review*, 26(2), pp.197–223

9. Miller, G. A., 1956. The Magical Number Seven, Plus or Minus Two: Some Limits on Our Capacity for Processing Information. *Psychological Review*, 63(2), pp.81–97

10. Cowan, N., 2001. The Magical Number 4 in Short-Term Memory: A Reconsideration of Mental Storage Capacity. *Behavioral and Brain Sciences*, 24(1), pp.87–114

11. Alloway, T. P. and Alloway, R. G., 2010. Investigating the predictive roles of working memory and IQ in academic attainment. *Journal of Experimental Child Psychology*, 106(1), pp.20–9

12. Sweller J., Van Merriënboer, J. J. G. and Paas F. 1998. Cognitive Architecture and Instructional Design. *Educational Psychology Review*, 10(3), pp.251–96

13. Ericsson, K. A. and Kintsch, W., 1995. Long-Term Working Memory. *Psychological Review*, 102(2), pp.211–45

14. Dochy, F., 1992. *Assessment of prior knowledge as a determinant for future learning: The use of prior knowledge state tests and knowledge profiles.* Utrecht/London: Lemma B. V./Jessica Kingsley Publishers

15. Willingham, D. T., 2009. *Why Don't Students Like School?: A Cognitive Scientist Answers Questions About How the Mind Works and What It Means for the Classroom.* San Francisco: John Wiley & Sons., p.110

16. Chi, M. T. H., 2006. Two Approaches to the Study of Experts' Characteristics. In Ericsson, K. A. et al., eds. *The Cambridge Handbook of Expertise and Expert Performance*, Cambridge UK: Cambridge University Press, pp.21–30

17. Kirschner P. A., Sweller J. and Clark R. E., 2006. Why Minimal Guidance During Instruction Does Not Work: An Analysis of the Failure of Constructivist, Discovery, Problem-Based, Experiential, and Inquiry-Based Teaching. *Educational Psychologist*, 41(2), pp.75–86

18. Rosenshine, B. and Stevens, R., 1986. Teaching Functions. In M. C. Wittrock, M. C., ed. *Handbook of Research on Teaching* (3rd ed.). Washington, DC: American Educational Research Association, pp.376–91

19. Przychodzin, A. M., Marchand-Martella, N. E., Martella, R. C. and Azim, D., 2004. Direct Instruction Mathematics Programs: An Overview and Research Summary. *Journal of Direct Instruction*, 4(1), pp.53–84

20. Morgan, P. L. et al., 2015. Which Instructional Practices Most Help First-Grade Students With and Without Mathematics Difficulties?. *Educational Evaluation and Policy Analysis*, 37(2), pp.184–205

21. Stebbins, L. B., 1977. *Education as Experimentation: A Planned Variation Model*, Volume 4(a). Lanham, MD: University Press of America

22. Adams, G. L. and Engelmann, S., 1996. *Research on Direct Instruction: 25 years beyond DISTAR.* Seattle, WA: Educational Achievement Systems

23. Mayer, R. E., 2004. Should There Be a Three-Strikes Rule Against Pure Discovery Learning?. *American Psychologist*, 59(1), pp.14–9

24. Ibid.

25. Ibid.

26. Ibid.

27. Geary, D. C., 1995. Reflections of Evolution and Culture in Children's Cognition: Implications for Mathematical Development and Instruction. *American Psychologist*, 50(1), pp.24–37

28. Hirsch, E. D., 2006. *The Knowledge Deficit: Closing the Shocking Education Gap for American Children.* Boston: Houghton Mifflin, pp.7–8

29. Sacks D., 2013. *Language Visible: Unravelling the Mystery of the Alphabet From A to Z.* Toronto: Alfred A Knopf, p.xiv

30. Miller G. A. and Gildea P. M., 1987. How Children Learn Words. *Scientific American,* 257(3), pp.94–9

31. Young, M., 2018. A knowledge-led curriculum: Pitfalls and possibilities. *Impact,* 4, pp.1–4

2: How can we use technology to personalize learning?

1. Herold, B., 2016. Personalized Learning: What Does the Research Say? *Education Week,* 36, pp.14–5

2. Summit Learning, 2019. *About T. L. P. Education* [online]. Available at <https://www.summitlearning.org/about-tlp> (accessed 4 November 2019)

3. Zuckerberg, M., 2017. Lessons in Philanthropy 2017. [Facebook]. 13 December. Available at <https://www.facebook.com/notes/mark-zuckerberg/lessons-in-philanthropy-2017/10155543109576634/> (accessed 4 November 2019)

4. Bloom, B. S., 1984. The 2 sigma problem: The Search for Methods of Group Instruction as Effective as One-to-One Tutoring. *Educational researcher,* 13(6), pp.4–16

5. Wiliam, D., 2015. Benjamin Bloom and the Two-Standard-Deviation Effect. *Learning Sciences Dylan Wiliam Center* [online]. Available at <https://www.dylanwiliamcenter.com/benjamin-bloom-and-the-two-standard-deviation-effect/> (accessed 3 November 2019)

6. Ander, R., Guryan, J. and Ludwig, J. 2016. *Improving Academic Outcomes for Disadvantaged Students: Scaling up Individualized Tutorials.* Report prepared for the Brookings Institute. Washington DC: Brookings Institute

7. Slavin, R. E. et al., 2011. Effective programs for struggling readers: A best-evidence synthesis. *Educational Research Review,* 6(1), pp.1–26

8. Wiliam, D., 2015 (see note 5)

9. Kraft, M. A., 2018. *Interpreting Effect Sizes of Education Interventions.* Working Paper. Brown University.

10. Slavin, R. E., 1987. Mastery Learning Reconsidered. *Review of Educational Research,* 57(2), pp.175–213

11. Pane, J. F., et al., 2017. *Informing Progress: Insights on Personalized Learning Implementation and Effects.* Santa Monica, CA: RAND corporation, p.6

12. Children Schools and Families Committee, National Curriculum, 2008. *Examination of Witnesses,* 17 November, London, UK: House of Commons Publications, Q505, Available at <https://publications.parliament.uk/pa/cm200809/cmselect/cmchilsch/344/8111704.htm> (accessed 4 November 2019)

13. Ibid., Q489

14. Macdonald, K. et al., 2017. Dispelling the Myth: Training in Education or Neuroscience Decreases but Does Not Eliminate Beliefs in Neuromyths. *Frontiers in Psychology,* 8, Article 1314. Available at <doi: 10.3389/fpsyg.2017.01314> (accessed 14 November 2019)

15. Pashler, H., McDaniel, M., Rohrer, D. and Bjork, R., 2009. Learning styles concepts and evidence. *Psychological Science in the Public Interest*, 9(3), pp.105–19

16. Coffield, F., Moseley, D., Hall, E. and Ecclestone, K., 2004. *Should We Be Using Learning Styles? What Research Has to Say to Practice*. London: Learning and Skills Research Centre

17. Kavale, K. A., Hirshoren, A. and Forness, S. R., 1998. Meta-analytic validation of the Dunn and Dunn model of learning-style preferences: A critique of what was Dunn. *Learning Disabilities Research and Practice*, 13, pp.75–80

18. Pashler, H., et al., 2009 (see note 15)

19. Ibid.

20. Willingham, D. T., 2005. Ask the Cognitive Scientist: Do Visual, Auditory, and Kinesthetic Learners Need Visual, Auditory, and Kinesthetic Instruction?. *American Educator*, 29(2). Available at <https://www.readingrockets.org/article/do-visual-auditory-and-kinesthetic-learners-need-visual-auditory-and-kinesthetic-instruction> (accessed 14 November 2019)

21. Mayer, R. E., 2014. Introduction to Multimedia Learning, in Mayer, R. E. (ed.), *The Cambridge Handbook of Multimedia Learning*. Cambridge: Cambridge University Press, pp.1–24

22. Caviglioli, O., 2018. *Dual Coding for Teachers*. Woodbridge, UK: John Catt Educational, p.7

23. Ibid.

24. Willingham, D. T., 2005 (see note 20)

25. Summit Learning. *What is Summit Learning?* [online]. Available at <https://www.summitlearning.org/approach/learning-experience> (accessed 3 November 2019)

26. Ibid.

27. McNeil, K., 2018. *Summit Learning Blog, A Student's Most Important Lesson: Learning How To Learn* [online]. Available at <https://blog.summitlearning.org/2018/01/personalised-learning/> (accessed 3 November 2019)

28. Kruger, J. and Dunning, D., 1999. Unskilled and Unaware of It: How Difficulties in Recognizing One's Own Incompetence Lead to Inflated Self-Assessments. *Journal of Personality and Social Psychology*, 77(6), pp.1121–134

29. Soderstrom, N. C. and Bjork, R. A., 2013. Learning versus performance, in Dunn, D. S. (ed), *Oxford bibliographies online: Psychology*. New York: Oxford University Press

30. Bjork, E. L. and Bjork, R. A., 2011. Making Things Hard on Yourself, But in a Good Way: Creating Desirable Difficulties to Enhance Learning, in Gernsbacher, M. A., Pew, R. W., Hough, L. M., Pomerantz, J. R. (eds), *Psychology and the Real World: Essays Illustrating Fundamental Contributions to Society*, New York, NY: Worth Publishers, pp.56–64

31. Karpicke, J. D., Butler, A. C. and Roediger, H. L., 2009. Metacognitive strategies in student learning: Do students practise retrieval when they study on their own?. *Memory*, 17(4), pp.471–79

32. Rohrer, D. and Taylor, K., 2006. The effects of overlearning and distributed practise on the retention of mathematics knowledge. *Applied Cognitive Psychology,* 20(9), pp.1209–224

33. Scheiter, K., 2014. The Learner Control Principle in Multi-Media Learning, in Mayer, R. E. (ed.), *The Cambridge Handbook of Multimedia Learning.* New York: Cambridge University Press, p.491

34. Ibid., p.496

35. Ibid., p.498

36. Ibid., p.497

37. NHS England, 2016. *Improving Outcomes Through Personalised Medicine.* Available at <https://www.england.nhs.uk/wp-content/uploads/2016/09/improving-outcomes-personalised-medicine.pdf> (accessed 3 November 2019)

38. Sleeman, D. and Brown, J. S., 1982. *Intelligent Tutoring Systems.* Cambridge, Massachusetts: Academic Press

39. Vanlehn, K., 2006. The Behavior of Tutoring Systems. *International Journal of Artificial Intelligence in Education,* 16(3), pp.227–65

40. Falmagne, J-C. et al., 1990. Introduction to Knowledge Spaces: How to Build, Test, and Search Them. *Psychological Review,* 97(2), pp.201–24

41. McGraw Hill Education ALEKS, 2017. *What makes ALEKS unique?* Available at <https://www.aleks.com/about_aleks/What_Makes_ALEKS_Unique.pdf> (accessed 3 November 2019)

42. Ritter, S. et al., 2007. Cognitive Tutor: Applied research in mathematics education. *Psychonomic Bulletin & Review,* 14(2), pp.249–55

43. Escueta, M., et al., 2017. *Education technology: an evidence-based review.* Working paper 23744. Cambridge, Massachusetts: National Bureau of Economic Research, pp.21–22

44. Ma, W., et al., 2014. Intelligent Tutoring Systems and Learning Outcomes: A Meta-Analysis. *Journal of Educational Psychology,* 106(4), pp.901–18

45. Steenbergen-Hu, S., and Cooper, H., 2013. A Meta-Analysis of the Effectiveness of Intelligent Tutoring Systems on K–12 students' Mathematical Learning. *Journal of Educational Psychology,* 105(4), pp.970–87

46. VanLehn, K., 2011. The Relative Effectiveness of Human Tutoring, Intelligent Tutoring Systems, and Other Tutoring Systems. *Educational Psychologist,* 46(4), pp.197–221

47. Cheung, A. and Slavin, R. E., 2012. *The Effectiveness of Educational Technology Applications for Enhancing Reading Achievement in K-12 Classrooms: A Meta-Analysis.* Baltimore, Maryland: Johns Hopkins University, Center for Research and Reform in Education

48. Cheung, A. and Slavin, R. E., 2013. The Effectiveness of Educational Technology Applications for Enhancing Mathematics Achievement in K-12 Classrooms: A Meta-Analysis. Baltimore, Maryland: Johns Hopkins University, Center for Research and Reform in Education

49. Smartick, 2019. Smartick and School. *Smartick* [online]. Available at <https://uk.smartickmethod.com> (accessed 4 November 2019)

50. Johanes, P. and Lagerstrom, L., 2017. *Adaptive Learning: The Premise, Promise, and Pitfalls.* Proceedings of the 124th ASEE Annual Conference and Exposition, Columbus, Ohio, 25–28 June

51. Escueta, M., et al., 2017 (see note 43)

3: Why can't we just look it up?

1. Vamvakitis, G., 2019. *Around the world and back with Google for Education* [online]. 29 January. Available at <https://www.blog.google/outreach-initiatives/education/around-the-world-and-back/> (accessed 3 November 2019)

2. Google for Education, 2019. *Teacher Center: Resources* [online]. Available at <https://teachercenter.withgoogle.com/resources/general> (accessed 4 November 2019)

3. Google for Education, 2019. *Teacher Center: Certification* [online]. Available at <https://teachercenter.withgoogle.com/certification_innovator> (accessed 4 November 2019)

4. Google for Education, 2019. *Search Education, Lesson Plans* [online]. Available at <https://www.google.com/insidesearch/searcheducation/lessons.html> (accessed 4 November 2019)

5. Glass, K. and Bergson-Michelson, T., 2012. 'Picking the Right Search Terms…'. [PowerPoint presentation]. *Beginner Lesson 1.* Updated by Russell, D. M., 2018. Available at <https://docs.google.com/presentation/d/1QbCY8VowB98NslEcorcbO9H R3Ef30tki3jJSHJuKErE/edit#slide=id.i0> (accessed 4 November 2019)

6. Google for Education, 2019. *Intermediate 1: Picking the right search terms* [online]. Available at <https://docs.google.com/document/d/1zZ6C6CN_51L9_TUIUjMJWf_yWfzAJzi8koZWVTuXxb0/edit> (accessed 4 November 2019)

7. Google for Education, 2019. *Advanced 1: Picking the right search terms* [online]. Available at <https://docs.google.com/document/d/10nYxhi3YfaVYJDHsXWHouxRmR AIN6UKpCNslJ0DU55k/edit> (accessed 4 November 2019)

8. Google for Education, 2019. *Beginner & Intermediate 5: Evaluating credibility of sources* [online]. Available at <https://docs.google.com/document/d/1wpDm3zSQn8xg fsM4k53MKXopO9YshbFp7og9LZmDN6Y/edit> (accessed 4 November 2019)

9. Google for Education, 2019. *Search Smart* [online]. Available at <https://teachercenter. withgoogle.com/fundamentals/unit?unit=51&lesson=53> (accessed 4 November 2019)

10. Ibid.

11. Google for Education, 2019. *Teacher Center Resource: How do you eat a cupcake?* [online]. Available at <https://teachercenter.withgoogle.com/resources/general/details? key=ahpzfmd3ZWltZWR1LXRyYWluaW5nLWNlbnRlcnIccCxlPR2VuZXJhbFJlc291cm NlGICAgMz12oIKDA> (accessed 4 November 2019)

12. Google for Education, 2019. *Teacher Center Resource: About Me with Google Slides* [online]. Available at <https://teachercenter.withgoogle.com/resources/general/ details?key=ahpzfmd3ZWltZWR1LXRyYWluaW5nLWNlbnRlcnIccCxlPR2VuZXJhbFJlc 291cmNlGICAgMz0yYwKDA> (accessed 4 November 2019)

13. Google for Education, 2019. *Teacher Center Resource: "If they had Twitter…"* [online]. Available at <https://teachercenter.withgoogle.com/resources/general/details?key=ahpzfmd3ZWItZWR1LXRyYWluaW5nLWNlbnRlcnIcCxIPR2VuZXJhbFJlc291cmNlGICAgLjZlZYJDA> (accessed 4 November 2019]

14. Simon H. and Chase W., 1973. Skill in Chess. *American Scientist.* 61(4), pp.394–403

15. Ibid.

16. Willingham, D. T., 2019. The Digital Expansion of the Mind Gone Wrong in Education. *Journal of Applied Research in Memory and Cognition,* 8(1), pp.20–4

17. Miller G. A. and Gildea P. M., 1987. How Children Learn Words. *Scientific American,* 257(3), pp.94–9

18. Ibid.

19. Hinds, P. J., 1999. The Curse of Expertise: The Effects of Expertise and Debiasing Methods on Prediction of Novice Performance. *Journal of Experimental Psychology: Applied,* 5(2), pp.205–21

20. Zapato, L., 2019. *Save the Pacific Northwest Tree Octopus,* Available at <https://zapatopi.net/treeoctopus/> (accessed 3 November 2019)

21. Pacific Northwest tree octopus, 2019. *Wikipedia.* Available at <https://en.wikipedia.org/wiki/Pacific_Northwest_tree_octopus> (accessed 3 November 2019)

22. Leu, D. and Castek, J., 2006. What Skills and Strategies are Characteristic of Accomplished Adolescent Users of the Internet?. *Annual Conference of the American Educational Research Association,* San Francisco, CA., April 7–11

23. Lumley, T. and Mendelovits, J., 2012. How well do young people deal with contradictory and unreliable information on line? What the PISA digital reading assessment tells us. *Australian Council for Educational Research* [online], p.3. Available at <http://research.acer.edu.au/pisa/3> (accessed 3 November 2019)

24. Ibid., p.4

25. Lewis, P., 2018. Fiction is outperforming reality: how YouTube's algorithm distorts truth. *The Guardian,* 2 February, Available at <https://www.theguardian.com/technology/2018/feb/02/how-youtubes-algorithm-distorts-truth> (accessed 3 November 2019)

26. Landrum, A. R. and Olshansky, A., 2019. YouTube as the Primary Propagator of Flat Earth Philosophy. Symposium at the American Association for the Advancement of Science (AAAS), February 14–7, Washington, DC

27. Hirsch, E. D., 2000. You Can Always Look It Up—or Can You? *American Educator,* 24(1), pp.4–9

28. Clark, R. C. and Mayer, R. E., 2016. *E-learning and the science of instruction: Proven guidelines for consumers and designers of multimedia learning.* [ebook] New Jersey: John Wiley & Sons. Available at <http://www.amazon.co.uk/kindlestore> (accessed 4 November 2019)

29. Mayer, R. E. (ed.), 2014. *The Cambridge Handbook of Multimedia Learning.* Cambridge: Cambridge University Press

30. Mayer, R. E., 2014. Introduction to Multimedia Learning, in Mayer, R. E. (ed). *The Cambridge Handbook of Multimedia Learning*. New York: Cambridge University Press, pp.1–24

31. Clark, R. C. and Mayer, R. E., 2016, (see note 28), loc. 2120–151

32. Ibid.

33. Ibid.

34. Butcher, K. R., 2014. The Multimedia Principle, in Mayer, R. E. (ed). *The Cambridge Handbook of Multimedia Learning*. New York: Cambridge University Press, pp.174–205

35. Chandler, P. and Sweller, J., 1991. Cognitive Load Theory and the Format of Instruction. *Cognition and Instruction*, 8(4), pp.293–332

36. Ibid.

37. Ibid.

38. Kalyuga, S. and Sweller, J., 2014. The Redundancy Principle in Multimedia Learning, in Mayer, R. E. (ed). *The Cambridge Handbook of Multimedia Learning*. New York: Cambridge University Press, pp.247–62

39. Mayer, R. E. and Pilegard, C., 2014. Principles for Managing Essential Processing in Multimedia Learning: Segmenting, Pre-training, and Modality Principles, in Mayer, R. E. (ed) *The Cambridge Handbook of Multimedia Learning*. New York: Cambridge University Press, pp.316–44

40. Van Gog, T., 2014. The Signaling (or Cueing) Principle in Multimedia Learning, in Mayer, R. E. (ed) *The Cambridge Handbook of Multimedia Learning*. New York: Cambridge University Press, pp.263–78

41. Mayer, R. E. and Logan F., 2014. Principles for Reducing Extraneous Processing in Multimedia Learning: Coherence, Signaling, Redundancy, Spatial Contiguity, and Temporal Contiguity Principles in Mayer, R. E. (ed) *The Cambridge Handbook of Multimedia Learning*. New York: Cambridge University Press, pp.279–315

42. Mayer, R. E., 2014, (see note 30), pp.2–3

43. Clark, R. C. and Mayer, R. E., 2016, (see note 28), loc. 2202

44. Oakley, B. A. and Sejnowski. T. J., 2019. What we learned from creating one of the world's most popular MOOCs. *npj Science of Learning*, 4, Article 7

45. Ibid.

46. Monbiot, G., 2017. In an age of robots, schools are teaching our children to be redundant. *The Guardian*, 15 February. Available at <https://www.theguardian.com/commentisfree/2017/feb/15/robots-schools-teaching-children-redundant-testing-learn-future> (accessed 4 November 2019)

47. Kaufman, J. C. and Baer, J., 2002. Could Steven Spielberg Manage the Yankees?: Creative Thinking in Different Domains. *The International Journal of Creativity & Problem Solving* 12(2), pp.5–14

48. Johnson, S., 2011. *Where Good Ideas Come from: The Natural History of Innovation*. London: Penguin, p.152

49. Ibid.

50. Cuban, L., 2015. Will teaching and learning become automated? Part 3. January 21. *Larry Cuban on School Reform and Classroom Practice* [online]. Available at <https://larrycuban.wordpress.com/2015/01/21/will-teaching-and-learning-become-automated-part-3/> (accessed 3 November 2019)

51. Murphy, T., 2011. MPG of a human. November 29. *You Do the Math* [online]. Available at <https://dothemath.ucsd.edu/2011/11/mpg-of-a-human/> (accessed 3 November 2019)

52. US Department of Energy, 2019. *All Electric Vehicles* [online]. Available at <https://www.fueleconomy.gov/feg/evtech.shtml> (accessed 3 November 2019)

4: How can we use technology to make learning active?

1. Futuresource Consulting, 2018. *K–12 Education Market Continues to Provide Growth Opportunities to PC OEMs and the Major OS Providers* [online]. Available at <https://futuresource-consulting.com/press-release/education-technology-press/k-12-education-market-continues-to-provide-growth-opportunities-to-pc-oems-and-the-major-os-providers/> (accessed 3 November 2019)

2. Microsoft 21st Century Learning Design, 2019. *Anchor Lessons: School Change* [online]. Available at <https://onedrive.live.com/redir?resid=91F4E618548FC604%21300&authkey=%21AOE-MnST_ZCMc1Q&page=View&wd=target%28Real-World%20Problem-Solving.one%7C70ddd634-c0d4-434d-a2c6-409b367c0ead%2FAnchor%20Lessons%7Cc90d384a-88fc-46a6-905a-ccf02a40dc8c%2F%29> (accessed 3 November 2019)

3. Microsoft 21st Century Learning Design, 2019. *Anchor Lessons: Mr Sun. E. Day* [online]. Available at <https://onedrive.live.com/redir?resid=91F4E618548FC604%21300&authkey=%21AOE-MnST_ZCMc1Q&page=View&wd=target%28Collaboration.one%7Ca1cfcdb9-1676-4a61-8c2c-090b5a07114a%2FAnchor%20Lessons%7Ca6f49c71-9c75-4dad-86b5-18884c33e20b%2F%29> (accessed 3 November 2019)

4. Microsoft Educator Center, 2019. *Problem-Based Learning: Module 7: Using Minecraft: Education Edition in problem-based learning* [online]. Available at <https://preview.education.microsoft.com/en-us/course/903e75a1/6> (accessed 3 November 2019)

5. Microsoft 21st Century Learning Design, 2019. *Anchor Lessons: Doing Business in Birmingham* [online]. Available at <https://onedrive.live.com/redir?resid=91F4E618548FC604%21300&authkey=%21AOE-MnST_ZCMc1Q&page=View&wd=target%28Skilled%20Communication.one%7C1afd7400-113e-4a39-89d3-f29aea4cf019%2FAnchor%20Lessons%7C2e8be5ff-5e52-4f0f-963a-994a7e950492%2F%29> (accessed 3 November 2019)

6. Apple, 2018. *Everyone Can Create: Teacher Guide* [online]. Available at <https://books.apple.com/book/id1357353934> (accessed 4 November 2019)

7. Apple, 2019. *Tools for Teaching* [online]. Available at <https://www.apple.com/uk/education/teaching-tools/> (accessed 4 November 2019)

8. Apple, 2018, (see note 6), p.16

9. Ibid., p.12

10. Ibid., p.17

11. Ibid., p.9

12. Ibid., p.8

13. Ibid., p.4

14. Kirschner P. A., Sweller J. and Clark R. E., 2006. Why Minimal Guidance During Instruction Does Not Work: an Analysis of the Failure of Constructivist, Discovery, Problem-Based, Experiential, and Inquiry-Based Teaching. *Educational Psychologist.* 41(2), pp.75–86

15. Willingham, D. T., 2009. *Why Don't Students Like School?: A Cognitive Scientist Answers Questions About How the Mind Works and What It Means for the Classroom.* San Francisco: John Wiley & Sons., p.61

16. Ibid., p.54

17. Singleton, C., Shear, L., Iwatani, E., Nielsen, N., House, A., Vasquez, S., Wetzel, T. and Gerard, S., 2018. *The Apple and ConnectED Initiative: Baseline and Year 2 Findings from Principal, Teacher, and Student Surveys.* Menlo Park, VA: SRI Education, p.1

18. Ibid., p.3

19. Ibid., p.5

20. Apple, 2018, (see note 6), p.i and p.iii

21. Koretz, D., 2017. *The Testing Charade: Pretending to Make Schools Better.* Chicago, Ill: University of Chicago Press

22. Roediger, H. L. and Karpicke, J. D., 2006. The Power of Testing Memory: Basic Research and Implications for Educational Practice. *Perspectives on Psychological Science*, 1(3), pp.181–210

23. Memrise, 2019. *Memrise, About Us* [online]. Available at <https://www.memrise.com/about/> (accessed 4 November 2019)

24. HegartyMaths, 2019. *Hegarty Maths* [online]. Available at <https://hegartymaths.com/> (accessed 4 November 2019)

25. Kuznekoff, J. H., Munz, S. and Titsworth, S., 2015. Mobile Phones in the Classroom: Examining the Effects of Texting, Twitter, and Message Content on Student Learning. *Communication Education*, 64(3). pp.344–65

26. Ebbinghaus, H., 1913. *Memory: A Contribution to Experimental Psychology.* Translated by H. A. Ruger and C. E. Bussenius. New York: Teachers College, Columbia University

27. Graph adapted from: Schimanke, F., Mertens, R. and Vornberger, O., 2014. Spaced repetition learning games on mobile devices: Foundations and perspectives. *Interactive Technology and Smart Education.* 11(3), pp.201–22

28. Cepeda, N. J., et al., 2006. Distributed practice in verbal recall tasks: A review and quantitative synthesis. *Psychological Bulletin.* 132(3), pp.354–80

29. Bjork, R. A., 1999. Assessing our own competence: Heuristics and illusions, in D. Gopher and A. Koriat (eds), *Attention and Performance XVII: Cognitive Regulation of Performance: Interaction of Theory and Application.* Cambridge, MA: MIT Press, pp.435–59

30. Dempster, F. N., 1988. The spacing effect: A case study in the failure to apply the results of psychological research. *American Psychologist.* 43(8), pp.627–34

31. Pashler, H. et al., 2007. Enhancing learning and retarding forgetting: Choices and consequences. *Psychonomic Bulletin & Review,* 14(2), pp.187–93

32. Storm, B. C., Bjork, R. A. and Storm, J. C., 2010. Optimizing retrieval as a learning event: When and why expanding retrieval practice enhances long-term retention. *Memory & Cognition,* 38(2), pp.244–53

33. Anki, 2019. *Anki 2.1 User Manual – What spaced repetition algorithm does Anki use?* [online]. Available at <https://apps.ankiweb.net/docs/manual.html#what-algorithm> (accessed 4 November 2019)

34. Harlow, I. M., Mumma, P. T and Smith Lewis, A., 2016. *Translating Learning Science into Learning Strategy, Cerego White Paper,* San Francisco: Cerego. Available at <https://cerego.com/pdf/Whitepaper.pdf> (accessed 4 November, 2019), p.22

35. Settles, B. and B. Meeder, B., 2016. A Trainable Spaced Repetition Model for Language Learning. *Proceedings of the 54th Annual Meeting of the Association for Computational Linguistics (Volume 1: Long Papers),* pp.1848–58

36. Ibid.

37. Cepeda, N. J., et al., 2006, (see note 28)

38. Ericsson K. A., Krampe R. T. and Tesch-Römer, C., 1993. The Role of Deliberate Practice in the Acquisition of Expert Performance. *Psychological Review,* 100(3), pp.363–406

39. Barton, C., 2018. Fractions and Decimals: Guess the Misconception. 13 February. *Eedi* [online]. Available at <https://medium.com/eedi/fractions-and-decimals-guess-the-misconception-65101c3dd993> (accessed 4 November 2019)

40. Anderson, J. R., Lynne M. R. and Simon, H. A., 2000. Applications and Misapplications of Cognitive Psychology to Mathematics Instruction. *Texas Education Review,* 1(2), pp.29–49

41. Maths Circle, 2019. *Times Tables Rock Stars* [online]. Available at <https://www.ttrockstars.com> (accessed 4 November, 2019)

42. Maths Circle, 2019. *NumBots* [online]. Available at <https://numbots.com> (accessed 4 November, 2019)

43. Wiliam, D., 2011. *Embedded Formative Assessment.* Bloomington, IN: Solution Tree Press, p.122

44. Engelmann, S. and Silbert, J., 2005. Expressive Writing 1. US: SRA/McGraw-Hill

45. Hamdan, N. et al., 2013. *The Flipped Learning Model: A white paper based on the literature review titled a review of flipped learning.* Flipped Learning Network, p.3

46. Akçayır, G. and Akçayır, M., 2018. The flipped classroom: A review of its advantages and challenges. *Computers & Education,* 126, pp.334–45

47. Fearn, H., 2016. Skills or knowledge: which is more important?. *Schools Week* [online]. Available at <https://schoolsweek.co.uk/the-many-skills-mistakes/> (accessed 4 November 2019)

5: How should we use smart devices?

1. Rawthorn, A., 2019. A Few Stumbles on the Road to Connectivity. *New York Times*. 19 December. Available at <https://www.nytimes.com/2011/12/19/arts/design/a-few-stumbles-on-the-road-to-connectivity.html?pagewanted=all> (accessed 4 November 2019)

2. Mitra, S., 2000. *Minimally Invasive Education for Mass Computer Literacy*. Conference on Research in Distance and Adult Learning in Asia, 21–25 June, Hong Kong

3. Futuresource Consulting, 2018. *K-12 Education Market Continues to Provide Growth Opportunities to PC OEMs and the Major OS Providers* [Press release]. 5 September. Available at <https://futuresource-consulting.com/press-release/education-technology-press/k-12-education-market-continues-to-provide-growth-opportunities-to-pc-oems-and-the-major-os-providers/> (accessed 4 November 2019)

4. Sanou, B., 2017. *ICT Facts and Figures 2017*. Geneva, CH: International telecommunications union. Available at <https://www.itu.int/en/ITU-D/Statistics/Documents/facts/ICTFactsFigures2017.pdf> (accessed 4 November 2019)

5. Silver, L., 2019. *Smartphone Ownership Is Growing Rapidly Around the World, but Not Always Equally*. Washington, DC: Pew Research Center. Available at <https://www.pewresearch.org/global/2019/02/05/smartphone-ownership-is-growing-rapidly-around-the-world-but-not-always-equally/> (accessed 4 November 2019)

6. Young, J. R., 2012. A Conversation With Bill Gates About the Future of Higher Education. *The Chronicle of Higher Education*. 25 June. Available at <https://www.chronicle.com/article/A-Conversation-With-Bill-Gates/132591> (accessed 4 November 2019)

7. Cristia, J., Ibarraran, P., Cueto,S., Santiago, A. and Severin, E., 2012. *Technology and Child Development: Evidence from the One Laptop Per Child Program* (IDB Working Paper No. IDB-WP-304). Washington, DC: Inter-American Development Bank

8. Escueta, M., et al., 2017. *Education Technology: An Evidence-Based Review* (NBER Working Paper No. 23744). Cambridge, MA: National Bureau of Economic Research, p.17

9. Arora, P., 2010. Hope-in-the-Wall? A digital promise for free learning. *British Journal of Educational Technology*, 41(5), pp.689–702

10. Warschauer, M., 2003. *Technology and Social Inclusion: Rethinking the Digital Divide*. Cambridge, MA: MIT Press, pp.1–2

11. McLuhan, M., 1994. *Understanding media: The extensions of Man*. Reprint. Cambridge, MA: The MIT Press, 1994, p.7

12. Kozma, R. B., 1994. Will Media Influence Learning? Reframing the Debate. *Educational Technology Research and Development*. 42(2), pp.7–19

13. Baron, N. S., 2015. Words Onscreen: *The Fate of Reading in a Digital World*. New York: Oxford University Press, p.19

14. Simon H. A., 1969. Designing Organizations for an Information-Rich World. Cited in: Greenberger, M. (1971), *Computers, Communication, and the Public Interest*, Baltimore, MD: The Johns Hopkins Press, pp.40–1

15. Wu, T., 2017. *The Attention Merchants: The Epic Scramble to Get inside Our Heads.* London, UK: Atlantic Books

16. Ibid.

17. The Economist, 2017. The battle for consumers' attention. *The Economist* [online]. 9 February. Available at <https://www.economist.com/special-report/2017/02/09/the-battle-for-consumers-attention> (accessed 4 November 2019)

18. Teixeira, T. S., 2014. *The Rising Cost of Consumer Attention: Why You Should Care, and What You Can Do About It. Harvard Business School.* Working Paper. pp.1–22

19. Helft, M. 2011. *The Class That Built Apps, and Fortunes. The New York Times* [online]. 8 May. Available at <https://www.nytimes.com/2011/05/08/technology/08class.html> (accessed 4 November 2019)

20. Duolingo, 2018. What is a streak? *Duolingo* [online]. Available at <https://support.duolingo.com/hc/en-us/articles/204980880-What-is-a-streak-> (accessed 4 November 2019)

21. BBC News, 2019. Snapchat under scrutiny from MPs over 'addictive' streaks'. *BBC* [online]. Available at <https://www.bbc.co.uk/news/technology-47623626> (accessed 4 November 2019)

22. Zeiler, M. D. and Price, A. E., 1965. Discrimination with Variable Interval and Continuous Reinforcement Schedules. *Psychonomic Science*, 3(1–12), p.299–300

23. Lewis, P., 2017. 'Our minds can be hijacked': the tech insiders who fear a smartphone dystopia. *The Guardian* [online]. 6 October. Available at <https://www.theguardian.com/technology/2017/oct/05/smartphone-addiction-silicon-valley-dystopia> (accessed 4 November 2019)

24. Lewis, P., 2018. 'Fiction is outperforming reality': how YouTube's algorithm distorts truth. *The Guardian* [online]. 2 February. Available at <https://www.theguardian.com/technology/2018/feb/02/how-youtubes-algorithm-distorts-truth> (accessed 4 November 2019)

25. Simonite, T., 2016. How Google Plans to Solve Artificial Intelligence. *MIT Technology Review* [online]. 31 March. Available at <www.technologyreview.com/s/601139/how-google-plans-to-solve-artificial-intelligence/>

26. Ofcom, 2018. *Children and parents: Media use and attitudes report 2018.* London, UK: Office of Communications. Available at <https://www.ofcom.org.uk/__data/assets/pdf_file/0024/134907/Children-and-Parents-Media-Use-and-Attitudes-2018.pdf> (accessed 4 November 2019), p.3

27. OECD, 2017. *PISA 2015 results (Volume III) Students' well-being.* Paris: OECD, pp.222–3. Available at <https://doi.org/10.1787/9789264273856-en> (accessed 4 November 2019)

28. Wallis, C., 2010. *The impacts of media multitasking on children's learning & development: Report from a research seminar.* New York, NY: The Joan Conney Center at Sesame Workshop, p.18

29. Ophir, E., Nass, C. and Wagner, A. D., 2009. Cognitive control in media multi-taskers. *Proceedings of the National Academy of Sciences,* 106(37), pp.15583–7

30. Jeong, S-H. and Hwang, Y., 2012. Does Multitasking Increase or Decrease Persuasion? Effects of Multitasking on Comprehension and Counterarguing. *Journal of Communication* 62(4), pp.571–87

31. Van Der Schuur, W. A., et al., 2015. The consequences of media multi-tasking for youth: A review. *Computers in Human Behavior.* 53, pp.204–15

32. Rideout, V. J.,. Foehr, G. U.and Roberts, D. F., 2010. *Generation M2: Media in the Lives of 8- to 18-Year-Olds.* Menlo Park, CA: Henry J. Kaiser Family Foundation, p.2

33. Yeykelis, L., Cummings, J. J. and Reeves, B., 2017. The Fragmentation of Work, Entertainment, E-Mail, and News on a Personal Computer: Motivational Predictors of Switching Between Media Content. *Media Psychology,* 21(3), pp.1–26

34. Van Der Schuur, W. A., et al., 2015, (see note 31)

35. Rosen, L. D., Carrier, M. L and Cheever, N. A., 2013. Facebook and texting made me do it: Media-induced task-switching while studying. *Computers in Human Behavior,* 29.3, pp.948–58

36. Rideout, V. J., 2015. *The Common Sense Census: Media Use by Tweens and Teens.* San Francisco, CA: Common Sense Media Incorporated, p.17

37. Burak, L. J., 2012. Multitasking in the University Classroom. *International Journal for the Scholarship of Teaching and Learning,* 6(2), pp.1–12

38. Kraushaar, J. M. and Novak, D. C., 2010. Examining the Affects of Student Multitasking with Laptops During the Lecture. *Journal of Information Systems Education,* 21(2), pp.241–51

39. Ravizza, S. M., Uitvlugt, M. G.and Fenn, K. M., 2017. Logged In and Zoned Out: How Laptop Internet Use Relates to Classroom Learning. *Psychological Science,* 28(2), pp.171–80

40. Prensky, M., 2001. Digital natives, digital immigrants part 1. *On the horizon,* 9(5), pp.1–6

41. Akçayır, M., Dündar, H. and Akçayır, G., 2016. What makes you a digital native? Is it enough to be born after 1980?. *Computers in Human Behavior,* 60, pp.435–40

42. Kirschner, P. A., and De Bruyckere, P., 2017. The myths of the digital native and the multi-tasker. *Teaching and Teacher Education,* 67, pp.135–42

43. Lui, D., Kirschner, P. A. and Karpinski, A. C., 2017. A meta-analysis of the relationship of academic performance and Social Network Site use among adolescents and young adults. *Computers in Human Behavior,* 77, pp.148–57

44. Willingham, D. T., 2010. Have Technology and Multi-tasking Rewired How Students Learn?. *American Educator,* 34(2)23, pp.24–8. Available at <https://www.aft.org/sites/default/files/periodicals/willingham-summer-10.pdf> (accessed 4 November 2019)

45. Hyman Jr, I. E., Benjamin A. S. and Wise-Swanson, B. M., 2014. Failure to see money on a tree: inattentional blindness for objects that guided behavior. *Frontiers in Psychology,* 5, Article 356

46. Laxmisan, A., Hakimzada, F., Sayan, O. R., Green, R. A., Zhang, J. and Patel, V. L., 2007. The multi-tasking clinician: Decision-making and cognitive demand during and after team handoffs in emergency care. *International Journal of Medical Informatics*, 76(11–12), pp.801–11

47. Ophir, E., et al.., 2009, (see note 29)

48. Brumby, D. P. and Salvucci, D. D., 2006. *Towards a Constraint Analysis of Human Multitasking*. Paper presented at the 7th International Conference on Cognitive Modeling, Trieste, Italy. 2006

49. Dux, P. E., et al., 2006. Isolation of a Central Bottleneck of Information Processing with Time-Resolved fMRI. *Neuron*, 52(6), pp.1109–20

50. Van Der Schuur, W. A., et al., 2015, (see note 31)

51. Carter, S. P., Greenberg, K. and Walker, M. S., 2017. The impact of computer usage on academic performance: Evidence from a randomized trial at the United States Military Academy. *Economics of Education Review*, 56, pp.118–32

52. Glass, A. L. and Kang, M., 2018. Dividing attention in the classroom reduces exam performance. *Educational Psychology*, 39(3), pp.395–408

53. Sana, F., Weston, T. and Cepeda, N. J., 2013. Laptop multitasking hinders classroom learning for both users and nearby peers. *Computers & Education*, 62, pp.24–31

54. Ward, A. F., et al., 2017. Brain Drain: The Mere Presence of One's Own Smartphone Reduces Available Cognitive Capacity. *Journal of the Association for Consumer Research* 2(2), pp.140–54

55. Oulasvirta, A., et al., 2012. Habits make smartphone use more pervasive. *Personal and Ubiquitous Computing*, 16(1), pp.105–14

56. Bosker, B., 2016. The Binge Breaker. *The Atlantic* [online]. November. Available at <https://www.theatlantic.com/magazine/archive/2016/11/the-binge-breaker/501122/> (accessed 4 November 2019)

57. Scheiter, K., 2014. The Learner Control Principle in Multi-Media Learning, in Mayer, R. E. (ed.), *The Cambridge Handbook of Multimedia Learning*. New York: Cambridge University Press

58. Carter, S. P., et al., 2017, (see note 51)

59. Glass, A. L. and Kang, M., 2018, (see note 52)

60. Beland, L-P. and Murphy, R., 2016. Ill communication: Technology, distraction & student performance. *Labour Economics*, 41, pp.61–76

61. Wilkinson, C., 2012. Shutting out a world of digital distraction. *The Telegraph* [online]. 6 September. Available at <https://www.telegraph.co.uk/culture/books/9522845/Shutting-out-a-world-of-digital-distraction.html> (accessed 4 November 2019)

6: The expertise of teaching: can technology help?

1. Shulman, L., 1987. Knowledge and Teaching: Foundations of the New Reform. *Harvard Educational Review.* 57(1), pp.1–23

2. Borko, H. and Livingston, C., 1989. Cognition and Improvisation: Differences in Mathematics Instruction by Expert and Novice Teachers. *American Educational Research Journal,* 26(4), pp.473–98

3. Clermont, C. P., Borko, H. and Krajcik, J. S., 1994. Comparative study of the pedagogical content knowledge of experienced and novice chemical demonstrators. *Journal of Research in Science Teaching,* 31(4), pp.419–41

4. Sabers, D. S., Cushing, K. S. and Berliner, D. C., 1991. Differences Among Teachers in a Task Characterized by Simultaneity, Multidimensional, and Immediacy. *American Educational Research Journal,* 28(1), pp.63–88

5. Kahneman, D. and Klein, G., 2009. Conditions for Intuitive Expertise: A Failure to Disagree. *American Psychologist,* 64(6), pp.515–26

6. Ibid.

7. Ericsson, K. A., 2006. The Influence of Experience and Deliberate Practice on the Development of Superior Expert Performance, in Ericsson, K. A., Charness, N., Hoffman, R. R. and Feltovich, P. J. (eds), *The Cambridge Handbook of Expertise and Expert Performance,* New York, NY: Cambridge University Press, pp.39–68

8. Hogan, T., Rabinowitz, M. and Craven III, J. A., 2003. Representation in Teaching: Inferences From Research of Expert and Novice Teachers. *Educational Psychologist,* 38(4), pp.235–47

9. Mr Barton Maths Blog, 2016. *Angle Facts – The Answers Revealed!* [online]. Available at <http://www.mrbartonmaths.com/blog/angle-facts-the-answers-revealed/> (accessed 21 November 2019)

10. Ofqual, 2015. *A Comparison of Expected Difficulty, Actual Difficulty and Assessment of Problem Solving across GCSE Maths Sample Assessment Materials.* Coventry, UK: Office of Qualifications and Examinations Regulation (Ofqual)

11. Hinds, P. J., 1999. The Curse of Expertise: The Effects of Expertise and Debiasing Methods on Prediction of Novice Performance. *Journal of Experimental Psychology: Applied,* 5(2), 205–21

12. Kahneman, D. and Klein, G., 2009, (see note 5)

13. Grossman, P., 1985. A passion for language: From text to teaching. *Knowledge Growth in Teaching Publications Series.* Stanford, CA: Stanford University, School of Education

14. Schempp, P. G., et al., 1998. Subject Expertise and Teachers' Knowledge. *Journal of Teaching in Physical Education,* 17(3), pp.342–56

15. Kahneman, D. and Klein, G., 2009, (see note 5)

16. Goldin, C. and Cecilia Rouse, C., 2000. Orchestrating Impartiality: The Impact of "Blind" Auditions on Female Musicians. *American Economic Review,* 90(4), pp.715–41

17. Kahneman, D. and Klein, G., 2009, (see note 5)

18. Baumeister, R. F. et al., 1998. Ego Depletion: Is the Active Self a Limited Resource?. *Journal of Personality and Social Psychology,* 74(5), pp.1252–65

19. Kahneman, D., 2011. *Thinking, Fast and Slow.* New York, NY: Macmillan, p.228

20. Ibid.

21. Howard, J. W., and Dawes, R. M., 1976. Linear Prediction of Marital Happiness. *Personality and Social Psychology Bulletin,* 2(4), pp.478–80

22. myFICO, 2019. *FICO Credit Score Estimator.* Available at <https://www.myfico.com/fico-credit-score-estimator/estimator> (accessed 4 November 2019)

23. Kahneman, D., 2011, (see note 19), p.227

24. Meehl, P. E., 1954. *Clinical Versus Statistical Prediction.* Minneapolis: University of Minnesota Press

25. Dawes, R. M., Faust, D. and Meehl, P. E., 1989. Clinical Versus Actuarial Judgment. *Science,* 243(4899), pp.1668–74

26. Christensen, C. M., Johnson, C. W. and Horn, M. B., 2010. *Disrupting Class.* New York: McGraw-Hill, p.98

27. Kuhl, P. K., Tsao, F.-M. and Liu, H-M., 2003. Foreign-language experience in infancy: Effects of short-term exposure and social interaction on phonetic learning. *Proceedings of the National Academy of Sciences,* 100(15), pp.9096–101

28. Meltzoff, A. N. et al., 2009. Foundations for a New Science of Learning. *Science,* 325(5938), pp.284–8

29. Collins, H., 2010. *Tacit and Explicit Knowledge.* Chicago, Ill: University of Chicago Press

30. Dunbar, R. I. M., 2016. Do online social media cut through the constraints that limit the size of offline social networks?. *Royal Society Open Science,* 3(1). Available at <https://doi.org/10.1098/rsos.150292> (accessed 21 November 2019)

31. Turkle, S., 2017. *Alone Together: Why we expect more from technology and less from each other.* London, UK: Hachette

32. Fumihide, T., Cicourel, A. and Movellan, J. R., 2007. Socialization between toddlers and robots at an early childhood education center. *Proceedings of the National Academy of Sciences,* 104(46), pp.17954–8

33. Sejnowski, T. J., 2018. *The Deep Learning Revolution.* [ebook] Cambridge, MA: MIT Press. Available at <http://www.amazon.co.uk/kindlestore> (accessed 4 November 2019), loc. 3995

34. James, K. H., and Engelhardt, L., 2012. The effects of handwriting experience on functional brain development in pre-literate children. *Trends in Neuroscience and Education,* 1(1), pp.32–42. Available at <http://www.sciencedirect.com/science/article/pii/S2211949312000038> (accessed 21 November 2019)

35. Mueller, P. A. and Oppenheimer, D. M., 2014. The Pen is Mightier than the Keyboard: Advantages of Longhand over Laptop Note Taking. *Psychological Science,* 25(6), pp.1159–68

36. OECD, 2016. *PISA 2015 results (Volume I) Excellence and equity in education.* Paris: OECD, p.226. Available at <https://doi.org/10.1787/9789264266490-en> (accessed 13 November 2019)

37. Hattie, J. *What Works Best in Education: The Politics of Collaborative Expertise.* Pearson, 2015, p.1

38. Ehrenberg, R. G. et al., 2001. Does Class Size Matter?. *Scientific American* 285(5) pp.78–85

39. Kovarik, B., 2015. *Revolutions in Communication: Media History from Gutenberg to the Digital Age.* New York: Bloomsbury, p.33

40. HegartyMaths, 2019. *Hegarty Maths* [online]. Available at <https://hegartymaths.com/> (accessed 4 November 2019)

41. Smartick, 2019. *Smartick* [online]. Available at <https://uk.smartickmethod.com> (accessed 4 November 2019)

42. Up Learn, 2019. *Up Learn* [online]. Available at <https://uplearn.co.uk> (accessed 4 November 2019)

43. Such as: Memrise, 2019. *Memrise* [online]. Available at <https://www.memrise.com> or Duolingo, 2018. *Duolingo* [online]. Available at <https://www.duolingo.com> (accessed 4 November 2019)

44. Such as: Cerego, 2018. *Cerego* [online]. Available at <https://www.cerego.com> (accessed 4 November 2019)

45. TL Editors, 2019. BBC Bitesize Partners with Cerego to Deliver Personalized Learning Programs. *Tech & Learning.* 31 January. Available at <https://www.techlearning.com/news/bbc-bitesize-partners-with-cerego-to-deliver-personalized-learning-programs> (accessed 4 November 2019)

46. Eedi, 2018. *Diagnostic Questions* [online]. Available at <https://diagnosticquestions.com> (accessed 4 November 2019)

47. Such as: *Anki,* 2019. Anki [online]. Available at <https://apps.ankiweb.net> or Quizlet, 2019. *Quizlet* [online]. Available at <https://quizlet.com/en-gb> (accessed 4 November 2019)

48. Such as: Smartick, Memrise or Duolingo, Hegarty Maths, Up Learn (see notes 40–3) or Maths Circle, 2019. Times Tables Rock Stars [online]. Available at <https://www.ttrockstars.com> (accessed 4 November 2019)

49. Such as: Anki or Quizlet (see note 47)

50. Use the Diagnostic Questions website for examples: Eedi, 2018. *Diagnostic Questions* [online]. Available at <https://diagnosticquestions.com> (accessed 4 November 2019)

51. Such as: Cerego (see note 44)

52. BESA, 2019. Key UK Education Statistics. *BESA* [online]. Available at <https://www.besa.org.uk/key-uk-education-statistics/> (accessed 4 November 2019)

53. OECD, 2015. *Students, Computers and Learning. Making the connection.* Paris: PISA, OECD Publishing, p.21. Available at <https://doi.org/10.1787/9789264239555-en> (accessed 13 November 2019)

54. Ibid., p.15

55. Kahneman, D., 2011, (see note 19), p.244

7: The expertise of assessment: can technology help?

1. White, E. (1984) cited in: Vaughan, C. (1991) Holistic assessment: What goes on in the rater's mind?, in Hamp-Lyons, L. (ed.), *Assessing Second Language Writing in Academic Contexts*. Norwood, N. J.: Ablex Publishing Corporation, pp.111–25

2. Rhead, S., Black, B. and Pinot de Moira, A., 2016. *Marking consistency metrics: 14 November 2016*. Coventry: OFQUAL

3. Harlen, W., 2004. *A systematic review of the evidence of reliability and validity of assessment by teachers used for summative purposes*. London: EPPI-Centre, Social Science Research Unit, Institute of Education, University of London

4. Shorrocks D., Daniels S., Staintone R. and Ring, K., 1993. *Testing and Assessing 6 and 7 year-olds: The Evaluation of the 1992 Key Stage 1 National Curriculum Assessment*. Final report of National Union of Teachers and School of Education, Leeds University. London: College Hill Press

5. Thomas S., Madaus G. F., Raczek A. E., Smees R. (1998). Comparing teacher assessment and the standard task results in England: the relationship between pupil characteristics and attainment. *Assessment in Education*, 5, pp.213–46

6. Burgess, S. and Greaves, E., 2013. Test scores, subjective assessment and stereotyping of ethnic minorities. *Journal of Labor Economics*, 31(3), pp.535–76

7. Campbell, T., 2015. Stereotyped at Seven? Biases in Teacher Judgement of Pupils' Ability and Attainment. *Journal of Social Policy*, 44(3), pp.517–47

8. Meadows, M., and Billington, L., 2005. A Review of the Literature on Marking Reliability (Report for National Assessment Agency). London: AQA, pp.23–5

9. Spear, M., 1996. The influence of halo effects upon teachers' assessments of written work. *Research in Education*, 56(10), pp.85–7

10. Meadows, M., and Billington, L., 2005, (see note 8), pp.25–7

11. Breland, H. M., 1977. Can multiple-choice tests measure writing skills? *College Board Review*, 103, pp.32–3

12. Wheadon, C., Whitehouse, C., Spalding, V., Tremain, K. and Charman, M., 2009. *Principles and Practice of On-Demand Testing*. Coventry: Ofqual, Available at <www.ofqual.gov.uk/files/2009-01-principles-practice-on-demand-testing.pdf> (accessed 5 November 2019)

13. Birdsall, M., 2011. *Implementing Computer Adaptive Testing to Improve Achievement Opportunities*. Coventry: Ofqual

14. Messick, S., 1996. Validity and washback in language testing. ETS Research Report Series *Language Testing*, 13(3), pp.241–56

15. Page, E. B., 1968. The Use of the Computer in Analyzing Student Essays. *International Review of Education*, 14(2), pp.210–25

16. Ibid.

17. Powers, D. E., Burstein, J. C., Chodorow, M., Fowles, M. E. and Kukich, K., 2001. Stumping e-rater: *Challenging the validity of automated essay scoring* (GRE Research). Princeton, NJ: Educational Testing Service. Available at <http://www.ets.org/Media/Research/pdf/RR-01-03-Powers.pdf> (accessed 5 November 2019)

18. Duhigg, C. 2009. What Does Your Credit Card Company Know About You? *New York Times Magazine*, 12 May. Available at <https://www.nytimes.com/2009/05/17/magazine/17credit-t.html> (accessed 13 November 2019)

19. Fry, H., 2018. *Hello World: How to be Human in the Age of the Machine*, loc. 482. [ebook] Transworld Digital. Available at <http://www.amazon.co.uk/kindlestore> (accessed 4 November 2019)

20. Ibid.

21. Woolley, S., 2017. How More Americans are Getting a Perfect Credit Score, August 2017, *Bloomberg* [online]. 14 August. Available at <https://www.bloomberg.com/news/features/2017-08-14/obsessives-have-cracked-the-perfect-fico-credit-score-of-850> (accessed 5 November 2019)

22. Citron, D. K. and Pasquale, F., 2014. The Scored Society: Due Process for Automated Predictions. *Washington Law Review*, 89, pp.1–34

23. Laming, D. R. J., 2004. *Human Judgment: The Eye of the Beholder*. London: Thomson Learning, p.9

24. No More Marking, 2019. Comparative Judgement Demo [online]. Available at <https://www.nomoremarking.com/demo2> (accessed 5 November 2019)

25. Thurstone, L. L., 1927. A Law of Comparative Judgment. *Psychological Review*, 34(4), pp.273–86

26. Ofqual, *Marking reliability studies 2017*. Coventry, UK: Ofqual. Available at <https://assets.publishing.service.gov.uk/government/uploads/system/uploads/attachment_data/file/759283/Marking_reliability_-_FINAL64494.pdf> (accessed 5 November 2019)

27. Christodoulou, D., 2017. Validity and primary writing assessments. *The No More Marking Blog* [online]. 21 October. Available at <https://blog.nomoremarking.com/validity-and-primary-writing-assessments-f301833f9262> (accessed 5 November 2019)

28. Ibid.

29. Qualifications and Curriculum Development Agency, 2010. *The National Curriculum: level descriptions for subjects*. London, UK: QCDA. Available at <http://dera.ioe.ac.uk/10747/> (accessed 5 November 2019)

30. Standards and Testing Agency, 2015. *2016 national curriculum assessments key stage 2: Interim teacher assessment frameworks at the end of key stage 2*. London: STA

31. Moskal, B. M. and Leydens, J. A., 2000. Scoring Rubric Development: Validity and Reliability. *Practical Assessment, Research & Evaluation*, 7(10), pp.71–81

32. Popham, W. J., 2005. The Instructional Consequences of Criterion-Referenced Clarity. *Educational Measurement: Issues and Practice*, 13(4), pp.15–8

33. Rezaei, A. and Lovorn, M., 2010. Reliability and Validity of Rubrics for Assessment Through Writing. *Assessing Writing*, 15(1), pp.18–39

34. Chang, H. and Cartwright, N. L., 2008. Measurement, in Psillos, S. and Curd, M. (eds), *The Routledge Companion to Philosophy of Science*, New York, NY: Routledge, pp.367–75

35. Domingos, P., 2015. *The Master Algorithm: How the Quest for the Ultimate Learning Machine Will Remake our World.* New York: Basic Books, p.5

36. Hurley, M. and Adebayo, J., 2016. Credit Scoring in the Era of Big Data. *Yale Journal of Law and Technology,* 18(1), pp.148–216

37. Leinweber, D. J., 2009. *Nerds on Wall Street: Math, Machines and Wired Markets.* Hoboken, New Jersey: John Wiley and Sons, p.138

38. Vigen, T., 2019. *Spurious Correlations.* Available at <http://tylervigen.com/view_correlation?id=359> (accessed 5 November 2019)

39. Siegel, E., 2013. *Predictive Analytics: The Power to Predict Who Will Click, Buy, Lie, or Die.* Hoboken, New Jersey, NJ: John Wiley & Sons, p.154

40. Babyak, M. A., 2004. What You See May Not Be What You Get: A Brief, Nontechnical Introduction to Overfitting in Regression-Type Models. *Psychosomatic Medicine,* 66(3), pp.411–21

41. Huysmans, J. et al., 2011. An empirical evaluation of the comprehensibility of decision table, tree and rule based predictive models. *Decision Support Systems,* 51(1), pp.141–154

42. Card, D., 2017. The "black box" metaphor in machine learning. *Towards Data Science* [online]. 15 July. Available at <https://towardsdatascience.com/the-black-box-metaphor-in-machine-learning-4e57a3a1d2b0> (accessed 3 November 2019)

Conclusion: Disrupting education

1. Vlaskovits, P., 2011. Henry Ford, Innovation, and That "Faster Horse" Quote. *Harvard Business Review.*29 August. Available at <https://hbr.org/2011/08/henry-ford-never-said-the-fast> (accessed 4 November 2019)

2. Isaacson, W., 2012. The Real Leadership Lessons of Steve Jobs. *Harvard Business Review,* 90(4), 92–102

3. Mayer, R. E., 2004. Should There Be a Three-Strikes Rule Against Pure Discovery Learning?. *American Psychologist,* 59(1), pp.14–9

Glossary

A-level General Certificate of Education Advanced Level tests – a qualification in a specific subject typically taken by school students aged 17–18 in England, Wales and Northern Ireland

AS-level Advanced Subsidiary level, an independent qualification encompassing the first year of an A-level qualification's content, typically taken by school students aged 16–17 in England, Wales and Northern Ireland

Adaptive learning systems Digital systems which adapt the content and questions a student sees based on their previous responses or interaction with the system

ALEKS Assessment and LEarning in Knowledge Spaces is a Web-based, artificially intelligent assessment and learning system from McGraw Hill Publishers

GCSE General Certificate of Secondary Education – a qualification in a specific subject typically taken by school students aged 15–16 in England, Wales and Northern Ireland

MOOC Massive Open Online Course

OECD Organisation for Economic Co-operation and Development, an intergovernmental economic organization with 36 member countries, responsible for running PISA tests

Ofqual The Office of Qualifications and Examinations Regulation – a non-ministerial government department that regulates qualifications, exams and tests in England

PEG Project Essay Grade, an automated essay marker developed in the 1960s

PISA Programme for International Student Assessment

RAND US think tank: Research ANd Development

Rubric Mark scheme or marking guidelines used to judge the quality of open-ended questions like essays

Bibliography

Amplify, Center for Early Reading, 2018. Learning to Read, A Primer, Part 2. *Amplify* [online]. Available at <https://go.info.amplify.com/hubfs/Primer%20II/Primer2_2018_Final.pdf> (accessed 4 November 2019).

Anderson, J. R., Reder, L. M. and Simon H. A., 2000, Summer. Applications and Misapplications of Cognitive Psychology to Mathematics Education. *Texas Education Review*, 1(2), pp.29–49. Available at <http://act-r.psy.cmu.edu/papers/misapplied.html> (accessed 12 November 2019).

Apple, 2018. *Everyone Can Create: Teacher Guide* [online]. Available at <https://books.apple.com/book/id1357353934> (accessed 4 November 2019).

Babbage, C., 2011. *Passages from the Life of a Philosopher.* Cambridge University Press, p.67.

Barton, C., 2018. Fractions and Decimals: Guess the Misconception. 13 February. *Eedi* [online]. Available at <https://medium.com/eedi/fractions-and-decimals-guess-the-misconception-65101c3dd993> (accessed 4 November 2019)

Beck, I. L., McKeown, M. G. and Kucan, L., 2013. *Bringing words to life: Robust vocabulary instruction.* New York, NY: Guilford Press.

Cahill, L., 2019. How to Create Google Forms Locked Mode Lessons. *MassCUE* [online]. 15 April. Available at <https://www.masscue.org/cyberconk12-2/> (accessed 3 November 2019).

Christensen, C. M., Johnson, C. W. and Horn, M. B., 2010. *Disrupting class: How Disruptive Innovation Will Change the Way the World Learns.* [ebook] New York: McGraw-Hill. Available at <http://www.amazon.co.uk/kindlestore> (accessed 4 November 2019).

Clark, R. E., 1983. Reconsidering research on learning from media. *Review of Educational Research*, 53(4), pp.445–59.

Coffield, F., Moseley, D., Hall, E. and Ecclestone, K., 2004. *Learning styles and pedagogy in post-16 learning. A systematic and critical review.* London, UK: The Learning and Skills Research Centre (LSRC).

Edsurge, 2016. *Decoding Adaptive.* London, UK: Pearson. Available at <http://d3e7x39d4i7wbe.cloudfront.net/static_assets/PearsonDecodingAdaptiveWeb.pdf> (accessed 3 November 2019).

Engelmann, S. and Colvin, G., 2006. *Rubric for Identifying Authentic Direct Instruction Programs.* Available at <http://www.zigsite.com/PDFs/rubric.pdf> (accessed 4 November 2019).

Google for Education, 2019. *Boost Student Research Skills* [online]. Available at <https://teachercenter.withgoogle.com/fundamentals/unit?unit=51&lesson=54> (accessed 4 November 2019).

Google for Education, 2019. *Search Smart* [online]. Available at <https://teachercenter.withgoogle.com/fundamentals/unit?unit=51&lesson=53> (accessed 4 November 2019).

Harlow, I. M., Mumma, P. T. and Smith Lewis, A., 2016. *Translating Learning Science into Learning Strategy, Cerego White Paper,* San Francisco: Cerego. Available at <https://cerego.com/pdf/Whitepaper.pdf> (accessed 4 November, 2019).

Hattie J., 2009. *Visible Learning: A Synthesis of Over 800 Meta-Analyses Relating to Achievement.* New York: Routledge.

Higgins, S., Beauchamp, G., and Miller, D., 2007. Reviewing the Literature on Interactive Whiteboards, *Learning, Media and Technology,* 32 (3), pp.213–25.

Hill, I., 2018. Student Voice: 3 Ways Summit Learning Benefits Me. *Summit Learning* [online]. 11 July. Available at <https://blog.summitlearning.org/2018/07/summit-learning-benefits/> (accessed 4 November 2019).

Kahneman, D. and Klein, G., 2009. Conditions for Intuitive Expertise: A Failure to Disagree. *American Psychologist,* 64(6), pp.515–26.

Kirschner P. A., Sweller, J. and Clark, R. E., 2006. Why Minimal Guidance During Instruction Does Not Work: An Analysis of the Failure of Constructivist, Discovery, Problem-Based, Experiential, and Inquiry-Based Teaching. *Educational Psychologist,* 41(2), June, pp.75–86.

Kruger, J. and Dunning, D., 1999. Unskilled and unaware of it: How difficulties in recognizing one's own incompetence lead to inflated self-assessments. *Journal of Personality and Social Psychology,* 77(6), pp.1121–34.

Lapowsky, I., 2015. What Schools Must Learn From LA's iPad Debacle, *WIRED,* 5 August. Available at <https://www.wired.com/2015/05/los-angeles-edtech/> (accessed 12 May 2019).

Lepkowska, D., 2007. No blood on their hands. *The Guardian,* 4 December, Available at <https://www.theguardian.com/education/2007/dec/04/link.link3> (accessed 1 November 2019).

Lumley, T. and Mendelovits, J., 2012. *How well do young people deal with contradictory and unreliable information on line? What the PISA digital reading assessment tells us.* Camberwell, AU: Australian Council for Educational Research ACEReSearch. Available at <http://research.acer.edu.au/pisa/3> (accessed 4 November 2019).

Mayer, M., 2010. How is the Internet Changing the Way You Think? *The Edge* [online]. Available at <https://www.edge.org/response-detail/11973> (accessed 4 November 2019).

McNeil, K., 2018. A Student's Most Important Lesson: Learning How To Learn. *Summit Learning* [online]. 4 January. Available at <https://blog.summitlearning.org/2018/01/personalized-learning/> (accessed 4 November 2019).

Microsoft 21st Century Learning Design, 2019. *Anchor Lesson – Doing Business in Birmingham* [online]. Available at <https://onedrive.live.com/redir?resid=91F4E618548FC604%21300&authkey=%21AOE-MnST_ZCMc1Q&page=View&wd=target%28Skilled%20Communication.one%7C1afd7400-113e-4a39-89d3-f29aea4cf019%2FAnchor%20Lessons%7C2e8be5ff-5e52-4f0f-963a-994a7e950492%2F%29> (accessed 4 November 2019).

Microsoft 21st Century Learning Design, 2019. *The Big Ideas – Real-World Problem-Solving and Innovation* [online]. Available at <https://onedrive.live.com/redir?resid=91F4E618548FC604%21300&authkey=%21AOE-MnST_ZCMc1Q&page=View&wd=target%28Real-World%20Problem-Solving.one%7C70ddd634-c0d4-434d-a2c6-409b367c0ead%2FThe%20Big%20Ideas%20-%20Real-World%20Problem-Solving%20%7C407d6199-e83d-494c-a055-d647a9a5c9cd%2F%29> (accessed 4 November 2019).

Miller G. A. and Gildea P. M., 1987. How Children Learn Words. *Scientific American, September;* 257 (3), pp.94–99.

Mitra, S., 2000. *Minimally Invasive Education for Mass Computer Literacy.* Conference on Research in Distance and Adult Learning in Asia, 21–25 June, Hong Kong.

Muralidharan, K., Singh, A. and Ganimian, A., 2019. Disrupting Education? Experimental Evidence on Technology-Aided Instruction in India. *American Economic Review,* 109(4), pp.1426–60.

Newport, C., 2016. *Deep work: Rules for Focused Success in a Distracted World.* [ebook] London: Hachette UK. Available at <http://www.amazon.co.uk/kindlestore> (accessed 4 November 2019).

Newport, C., 2019. *Digital Minimalism: Choosing a Focused Life in a Noisy World.* London: Penguin UK.

OECD, 2016. *PISA 2015 Results (Volume II): Policies and Practices for Successful Schools,* Paris: OECD Publishing. Available at <http://dx.doi.org/10.1787/9789264267510-en> (accessed 4 November 2019).

OLPC News, 2010. *New Negropontism: You Can Give Kids XO Laptops and Just Walk Away* [online]. 22 December. Available at <http://www.olpcnews.com/people/negroponte/new_negropontism_you_can_give_kids_xo_laptops.html> (accessed 4 November 2019).

Pane, J. F. et al., 2017. *Informing Progress: Insights on Personalized Learning Implementation and Effects.* Santa Monica, CA: RAND Corporation.

Plant, E. A. et al., 2005. Why study time does not predict grade point average across college students: Implications of deliberate practice for academic performance. *Contemporary Educational Psychology*, 30 (1), pp.96–116.

Platt, K., 2019. What Is Personalized Learning (and What Isn't) with Summit Learning? *Summit Learning* [online]. 27 February. Available at <https://blog.summitlearning.org/2019/02/what-is-and-what-isnt-personalized-learning/> (accessed 4 November 2019).

Polanyi, M., 2012 ed. *Personal Knowledge*. Abingdon, UK: Routledge.

Polanyi, M., 1966. The Logic of Tacit Inference. *Philosophy*, 41(155), pp.1–18.

Postman, N., 1985. *Amusing Ourselves to Death: Public Discourse in the Age of Show Business*. New York, NY: Penguin.

Prensky, M., 2001. Digital Natives, Digital Immigrants Part 1. *On the Horizon*, 9(5), pp.1–6.

Simon, H. A., 1969. Designing Organizations for an Information-Rich World. Cited in: Greenberger, M. (1971), *Computers, Communication, and the Public Interest*, Baltimore, MD: The Johns Hopkins Press.

Singer, N., 2017. How Google Took Over the Classroom. *The New York Times*, 13 May. Available at <https://www.nytimes.com/2017/05/13/technology/google-education-chromebooks-schools.html> (accessed 3 November 2019).

Smith, F. J., 1913. The Evolution of the Motion Picture, *New York Dramatic Mirror*, 9 July, p.24.

Summit Learning, 2017. *The Science of Summit* [online]. Available at <https://summitps.org/wp-content/uploads/2018/09/The-Science-of-Summit-by-Summit-Public-Schools_08072017-1.pdf> (accessed 3 November 2019).

VanLehn, K. et al., 2005. The Andes Physics Tutoring System: Lessons Learned. *International Journal of Artificial Intelligence in Education*, 15(3), pp.147–204.

Wardrop, M., 2008. Learning by heart is 'pointless for Google generation'. *The Telegraph*, 2 December, Available at <www.telegraph.co.uk/education/primaryeducation/3540852/Learning-by-heart-is-pointless-for-Google-generation.html> (accessed 3 July 2019).

Wiliam, D., 2011. *Embedded Formative Assessment*. Bloomington, IN: Solution Tree Press.

Willingham, D. T., 2005. Ask the Cognitive Scientist: Do Visual, Auditory, and Kinesthetic Learners Need Visual, Auditory, and Kinesthetic Instruction? *American Educator*, 29(2). Available at <https://www.aft.org/ae/summer2005/willingham> (accessed 13 November 2019).

Willingham, D. T., 2007. Critical thinking. *American Educator*, 31, pp.8–19.

Willingham, D. T. and Daniel, D., 2012. Teaching to what students have in common. *Educational Leadership*, 69(5), pp.16–21.

Willingham, D. T., 2009. *Why Don't Students Like School?: A Cognitive Scientist Answers Questions About How the Mind Works and What It Means for the Classroom*. San Francisco: John Wiley & Sons.

Wolfe, T., 1967. Suppose he Is what he sounds like, the most important thinker since Newton, Darwin, Freud, Einstein, and Pavlov – what If he is right?, in Stearn, G. E. (ed.), *McLuhan: Hot & Cool,* New York, NY: The Dial Press.

Zuckerberg, M., 2015. A Letter to our daughter, Facebook, 1 December. Available at <https://en-gb.facebook.com/notes/mark-zuckerberg/a-letter-to-our-daughter/10153375081581634/> (accessed 4 November 2019).

Copyright acknowledgements

We are grateful to the authors and publishers for use of extracts from their titles and in particular for the following:

Barton, C., 2018: extracts and diagram from 'Fractions and Decimals: Guess the Misconception', 13 February. *Eedi*. Available at <https://medium.com>. AQA material is reproduced by permission of AQA.

Cahill, L., 2019: extracts from 'How to Create Google Forms Locked Mode Lessons', <engageducate.com>, 25 January. Reproduced by permission.

Caviglioli, O., 2018: extract and image from *Dual Coding for Teachers*. John Catt publishers. Reproduced by permission of the publisher and the author.

Chandler, P. and Sweller, J., 1991: extract and diagrams from 'Cognitive Load Theory and the Format of Instruction'. *Cognition and Instruction* 8(4), pp.293–332. Reprinted by permission of the publisher, Taylor & Francis Ltd <http://www.tandfonline.com>

Clark, R. C. and Mayer, R. E., 2016: extract and diagram from *E-learning and the science of instruction: Proven guidelines for consumers and designers of multimedia learning*. John Wiley & Sons. Permission granted via RightsLink.

Clark, R. E., 1983. 'Reconsidering research on learning from media' *Review of Educational Research* 53(4): pp.445–59 <https://doi.org/10.3102/00346543053004445> American Educational Research Association. Reproduced by permission of Sage Journals.

Christensen, C. M., Johnson, C. W. and Horn, M. B., 2010: *Disrupting class*. McGraw-Hill Education. Copyright © Clayton M. Christensen. Republished with permission of McGraw-Hill Education. Permission conveyed through Copyright Clearance Center.

Coffield, F., Moseley, D., Hall, E. and Ecclestone, K.: *Learning styles and pedagogy in post-16 learning. A systematic and critical review*. The use of 53 (fifty-three) words from London: Learning and Skills Research Centre. Reproduced by permission of Professor Frank Coffield.

EdSurge, 2016: *Decoding Adaptive*, London: Pearson. Copyright 2016. This work is licensed under the Creative Commons Attribution 4.0 International Licence <wwwcreativecommons.org/licenses>

Engelmann, S. and Colvin, G., 2006: *Rubric for identifying Authentic Direct Instruction Programs*, p.37 Copyright © S. Engelmann. Reproduced by permission of Engelmann-Becker Corporation.

Greenberger, Martin: *Computers, Communications and the Public Interest*. pp.29–30. Copyright © 1971 Martin Greenberger. Reprinted with permission of Johns Hopkins University Press.

Guardian Staff, 2007: No blood on their hands. *The Guardian*, 4 December <www.theguardian.com> Courtesy of Guardian News & Media Ltd.

Harlow, I. M., Mumma, P. T. and Smith Lewis, A.: extract and image from, *Translating Learning Science into Learning Strategy, Cerego White Paper*, p.22 <https://cerego.com/pdf> Reproduced by permission.

Hattie, J., 2009: *Visible Learning: A Synthesis of Over 800 Meta-Analyses Relating to Achievement*. New York, Routledge, Copyright © Christian Education, reprinted by permission of Informa UK Limited, trading as Taylor & Francis Group <www.tandfonline.com> on behalf of Christian Education.

Hirsch, E. D., 2000: 'You Can Always Look It Up—or Can You?' *American Educator* 24(1): pp.4–9. Used by permission of the Core Knowledge® Foundation.

Kruger, J. and Dunning, D., 1999: 'Unskilled and unaware of it: How difficulties in recognizing one's own incompetence lead to inflated self-assessments'. *Journal of Personality and Social Psychology*, 77(6), p.1121, published by American Psychological Association. Reprinted with permission.

Lumley, T. and Mendelovits, J., 2012: *How well do young people deal with contradictory and unreliable information on line? What the PISA digital reading assessment tells us*. <https://research.acer.edu.au/pisa/3>. Reproduced by permission of The Australian Council for Educational Research Ltd.

Miller G. A. and Gildea P. M., 1987: 'How Children Learn Words'. *Scientific American*; 257(3), pp.94–99, pp.97–98. Reprinted by permission of *American Scientist*, magazine of Sigma Xi, The Scientific Research Honor Society.

Muralidharan, K., Singh, A. and Ganimian, A., 2019: 'Disrupting Education? Experimental Evidence on Technology-Aided Instruction in India'. *American Economic Review*, 109(4). Copyright American Economic Association; reproduced with permission of the *American Economic Review*.

Negroponte, N.: extract from 'You Can Give Kids XO Laptops and Just Walk Away', *OLPC News*, 22 December <www.olpcnews.com> Creative Common Licence Attribution 3.0 <https://creativecommons.org>

Newport, C. 2019: The use of 53 (fifty-three) words from *Digital minimalism: Choosing a Focused Life in a Noisy World*, (Portfolio Penguin, 2019). First published in the United States of America by Portfolio/Penguin, an imprint of Penguin Random House LLC 2019. First published in Great Britain by Penguin Business, 2019. Copyright © Calvin C. Newport, 2019. Reproduced by permission of Penguin Books Ltd and Portfolio, an imprint of Penguin Publishing Group, a division of Penguin Random House LLC. All rights reserved.

Wiliam, D., 2011: *Embedded Formative Assessment*, pp.120 and 122. Bloomington, Solution Tree Press. Copyright © 2011 by Solution Tree Press. All rights reserved. Reproduced by permission.

Willingham, D. T., 2009: *Why Don't Students Like School?: A Cognitive Scientist Answers Questions About How the Mind Works and What It Means for the Classroom.* San Francisco: Jossey-Bass. John Wiley and Sons. Copyright © 2009 Daniel T. Willingham. All rights reserved.

Willingham, D. T., 2005: 'Ask the Cognitive Scientist Do Visual, Auditory, and Kinesthetic Learners Need Visual, Auditory, and Kinesthetic Instruction?' *American Educator*, 29(2), pp.8–19. Reprinted with permission from the Summer 2005 issue of *American Educator*, the quarterly journal of the American Federation of Teachers, AFL-CIO and the author.

Willingham, D. T., 2007: 'Critical thinking', *American Educator*, 31, p.8. Reprinted with permission from the Summer 2007 issue of *American Educator*, the quarterly journal of the American Federation of Teachers, AFL-CIO and the author.

Willingham, D. T. and Daniel, D., 2012: 'Teaching to what students have in common', *Educational Leadership*, 69(5), pp.16–21. Republished with permission of Assn for Supervision and Curriculum Development. Permission conveyed through Copyright Clearance Center, Inc.

'Mars! 22 March', extract and image from: Christodoulou, D., 2017. Validity and primary writing assessments. *The No More Marking Blog.* 21 October. <https://blog.nomoremarking.com> Reproduced by permission.

'One Sunny evening a gang called FG…' extract and image from: Christodoulou, D., 2017. Validity and primary writing assessments. *The No More Marking Blog.* 21 October. <https://blog.nomoremarking.com> Reproduced by permission.

Acknowledgements

Many people helped me write this book.

Nick Rose, Barbara Oakley, Maria Egan, Amanda Spielman, Harry Fletcher-Wood, Heather Fearn, Matthew Hanney, Jasper Green, Jonny Porter, Josh Perry, Katharine Birbalsingh, Michelle Major, Paul Kirschner, Christine Counsell, Clare Sealy, Flora Spielman and Polly Spielman offered advice and comments on early drafts, for which I am very grateful.

I am also grateful to Colin Hegarty, Ed Cooke, Bruno Reddy, Kris Boulton, Will Orr-Ewing, Andrew Smith Lewis and Daniel González de Vega for illuminating insights into their work.

Dr Chris Wheadon and all my colleagues at No More Marking have been a constant source of inspiration.

Paul Repper and the team at Oxford University Press, Olivia West and Oliver Caviglioli have provided wonderful editing, design and illustrations.

Any mistakes that remain are my own.

About the author

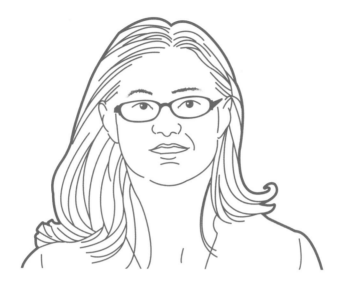

Daisy Christodoulou is the Director of Education at No More Marking, a provider of online comparative judgement. She works closely with schools on developing new approaches to assessment.

Before that, she was Head of Assessment at Ark Schools, a network of academy schools in England. She has taught English in two London comprehensives and has been part of government commissions on the future of teacher training and assessment.

Daisy is the author of *Seven Myths About Education* (2014) and *Making Good Progress? The future of Assessment for Learning* (2017).